Pacifiers Anonymous:

How to **Kick** the Pacifier or Thumb Sucking Habit

Pacifiers Anonymous:

How to **Kick** the Pacifier or Thumb Sucking Habit

Sumi Makkar Sexton, MD
Ruby Natale Andrew, PhD, PsyD
Liza Draper

MILL CITY PRESS | Minneapolis

Copyright © 2010 by Sumi Makkar Sexton, MD, Ruby Natale Andrew, PhD, PsyD, Liza Draper

Mill City Press, Inc.
212 3rd Avenue North, Suite 290
Minneapolis, MN 55401
612.455.2294
www.millcitypublishing.com

All rights reserved. No part of this publication may be reproduced, stored in a retrieval system, or transmitted, in any form or by any means, electronic, mechanical, photocopying, recording, or otherwise, without the prior written permission of the author.

ISBN - 978-1-936400-15-7
ISBN - 1-936400-15-4
LCCN - 2010932518

Cover Design & Typeset by Kristeen Wegner
Illustrations by Joe Jamaldinian

Printed in the United States of America

Acknowledgements

Words cannot describe how grateful we are for our loving children whose trials and tribulations inspired this book. This book would not have been possible without them. We are also grateful to our husbands for their support and continuous encouragement. In addition, we thank Mark Levine for his guidance and the staff members at Mill City Press who permitted us to publish this book.

About the Authors

Sumi Makkar Sexton, MD

Dr. Sumi Makkar Sexton is an assistant professor of family medicine at Georgetown University School of Medicine, Washington DC, and is a founding partner and President of Premier Primary Care Physicians in Arlington, Virginia (www.premierprimarycare.com). She is also an associate editor for *American Family Physician*, the best-read journal in the field of primary care. Dr. Sexton received her medical degree from the University of Miami School of Medicine in 1996 and completed a residency in family medicine at Georgetown University School of Medicine in 1999. She sees patients of all ages with a special interest in newborn care and children's health. She is often the physician for both children and their parents, which provides countless opportunities for counseling on health habits including pacifier and thumb sucking. She has written an article on the health effects of the pacifier published on April 15, 2009. Her writing and research in the field of pacifier and thumb sucking was not only fueled by her current medical practice, but also by her two young daughters, who were avid pacifier users.

Ruby Natale Andrew, PhD, PsyD

Dr. Ruby Natale Andrew is a practicing clinical child psychologist in Miami with expertise in early childhood development. She received her dual PhD and PsyD doctorate degrees from Nova Southeastern University, Ft. Lauderdale, Florida in 2000, and completed a fellowship in pediatric psychology at the University of Miami School of Medicine in 2003. She has extensive research and writing experience in the field of child psychology and has published several articles on topics including obesity, child abuse, and brain injury. Her research received national media attention in March 2008 and lead to both television and media interviews on *The Early Show*, local and national ABC news programs, *Washington Post*, etc. She has presented at numerous conferences nationwide. Dr. Natale Andrew is also a working mother of one daughter. Her interest in the field of pacifiers started when she had concerns about the pacifier's effect on breastfeeding her daughter.

Liza Draper

Liza Draper is a stay-at-home mom of two. Prior to having children, Liza was a writer for an art gallery and a social justice nonprofit organization. She has a BA from Bucknell University with a double major in history and the classics, providing her insight and interest in the history of pacifier and thumb sucking and cultural differences. She belongs to numerous mothering groups and online parent groups, and actively participates in parenting listserves, blogs, and Web sites.

Foreword

Before reading further, there are some unique features about this book you should know. First, we have three authors with three different view points: a physician, a child psychologist, and a full-time mom. Whenever each of us has a personal view to share based upon our professional or personal experiences, you will see our designated icon (see below). Also, the word "thumb" is used throughout the book to mean sucking on either a thumb or finger(s), or any part of the hand really. Most importantly, you'll soon notice that this book is a twelve-step guide with concrete solutions on how to kick the habit. This is different from other well-known twelve-step programs in that we are discussing a habit that is not necessarily dangerous or life-threatening. However, it is still a stress-provoking habit that has been a hot topic among parenting blogs, parenting books, and conversations in everyday life.

Dr. Sumi says:

As a family physician, a former pacifier addict, and the mother of two recently raging pacifier users, I am fascinated by the pacifier and the thumb and the way they captivate their users. I wanted to write this book to answer my own questions, along with common questions asked by my patients and fellow parents. Is sucking on the pacifier or thumb just an overindulgent behavior, or are there actually some benefits? Is it better to suck the pacifier or the thumb? When and how do you wean?

My first and last memory of my pacifier was my parents explaining that the zebra at the zoo took my pacifier when I was about two-and-a-half years old. I vaguely remember sadly repeating day after day "the zebra took my pacifier," until it eventually became an empty statement about an event that happened in my childhood. It wasn't until fifth grade when I drew a zebra stealing my pacifier for art class that I realized the truth about my beloved pacifier and my parents' plot against me. The plot continued when my mother said she knew from day one that each of her granddaughters loved to suck just as much as their mother did. For baby number one, I tried my hardest to resist, despite my mother's chanting, "You know she wants that pacifier!" For baby number two, I knew it was a hopeless case. A few years ago I was frantically looking on the Internet for a real guide to tell me I wasn't a bad parent for using the pacifier in the first place and how I could end the madness. To my surprise, there wasn't much out there aside from an article here or there or a small chapter in more general parenting books. From talking to my own patients in the office, I knew there were other parents out there with the same questions I had, and so my research in the field began…

Dr. Ruby says:

I am a clinical child psychologist, and my specialty area is early childhood development for children birth through age five. While many sometimes wonder if a "baby" really needs to see a psychologist, I urge them to consider all of the problems parents have with young children, like sleeping, feeding issues, behavior problems, tantrums, toilet training, and, yes, pacifier and thumb use! My role as a psychologist is to focus on giving parents the tools to better address children's issues like these. In my experience, many parents have problems weaning their children. The two main questions I am asked are 1) how do I wean? and 2) how do I get my child to sleep now that he does not have the pacifier or thumb to rely on anymore? Both of these areas are addressed in this book. I also have a young child of my own and, given all the problems I heard tied to pacifier use, I tried not to let her use one. As a result, I had a child who was not addicted to pacifiers but who had lots of trouble falling asleep at night and who has been difficult to wean from the breast (i.e., human pacifier). Therefore, in this book we address alternative soothing strategies for parents once they wean their children whether it's from the pacifier, thumb, or even other behaviors like breastfeeding.

Mommy Liza says:

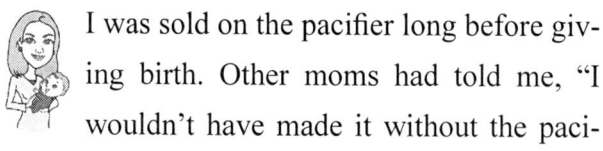

I was sold on the pacifier long before giving birth. Other moms had told me, "I wouldn't have made it without the pacifier," and "It's the only thing that stopped my baby from crying." As if that's not enough persuasion, I read that pacifiers reduce the risk of SIDS, and this paranoid mommy-to-be ran out and stocked up.

To my shock (and slight dismay), my newborn would have nothing to do with the pacifier. He sucked on it casually for the first week of life before spitting it out once and for all. What could be wrong? I tried different pacifier brands, shapes, and textures, dipped the pacifier in breast milk and stood over my baby while he slept, popping it back in each time he spat it out. Finally I gave up (after buying a SIDS baby monitor).

Pacifiers Anonymous intrigued me in part because of my interest in anthropology and human behavior. Why do some babies like to suck while others don't? Why do some continue to suck into childhood and seem to *need* their paci like I *need* my morning coffee? More importantly, though, this book interests me because I know how much help we parents need. As a stay-at-home mom (or, now that I have an active toddler, a "stay-*out*-of-the-home" mom), I've seen lots of pacifier battles. I can really empathize with the frustration these parents feel, having struggled myself with many other parenting issues. My struggles always lead me to parenting books. I would have been sunk without resources on breastfeeding, sleeping through the night, napping during the day, and toddler disciplining. Parents need a good resource to help them understand pacifier use and thumb sucking, and to help them make a clean break when they're ready. I hope this book is just that.

Step 1

Admitting the Addiction: Who loves it more— you or your little one?

Addiction sounds like such a harsh word, so if you're wondering if you're reading the right book, ask yourself these questions: Does your child have an obsession with the pacifier or thumb and crave it like you crave your morning coffee? Does it sometimes feel like he or she uses it uncontrollably? Are you afraid that stopping the pacifier or thumb could lead to anxiety, mood changes, or sleeplessness? That's addiction, my friend!

All joking aside, addiction experts might argue that if the action is not truly harmful, it might just be a compulsive behavior instead. Either way, it's a perfect setup for a twelve-step program to help kick the habit. Whether you are looking for some savvy rehab advice for your little pacifier or thumb lover, or if you are just wondering about the pros and cons of each, you've found the right book.

Roughly 75 to 90 percent of all infants suck a pacifier or thumb. In the past, the thumb was the sucking method of choice, but currently in the United States, the pacifier has made its way to *numero uno,* with user estimates as high as 74 percent. One study found that 20 percent of children sucked a pacifier beyond age three! Children who are pacifier lovers have been affectionately referred to as "paddicts" (pacifier addicts) among parenting bloggers. Other names for the pacifier include binky, dummy, nuk or nukky, and soother among dozens of other pet names. Thumb suckers are a bit different from their paddict pals in that they tend to suck into and beyond the toddler years since it can't just be "taken away." So by age three, the trend reverses, with more thumb suckers than pacifier suckers. In either the pad-

Admitting the Addiction

dict or thumb sucker's case, both lead to a habit that can be stress-provoking for both the parent and the child.

As parents, we probably know that we too can benefit from the pacifier or thumb. After all, doesn't a happy child equal a happy parent? And who doesn't appreciate a peaceful night's sleep? We become "enablers" of this so-called addiction. We gave a pacifier to our little one in the first place, sometimes after much struggle to find the exact pacifier model that did the trick. Or we gently helped them find their fingers to suck on and were relieved when they found them on their own. Whether we've encouraged the pacifier or the thumb, each can lead to a habit that is equally hard if not harder for the parents to break. Sometimes the habit just gives us that edge we need to get through a busy day or a tough work schedule or a move to a new home or the birth of another child or even just everyday life.

Dr. Sumi says:

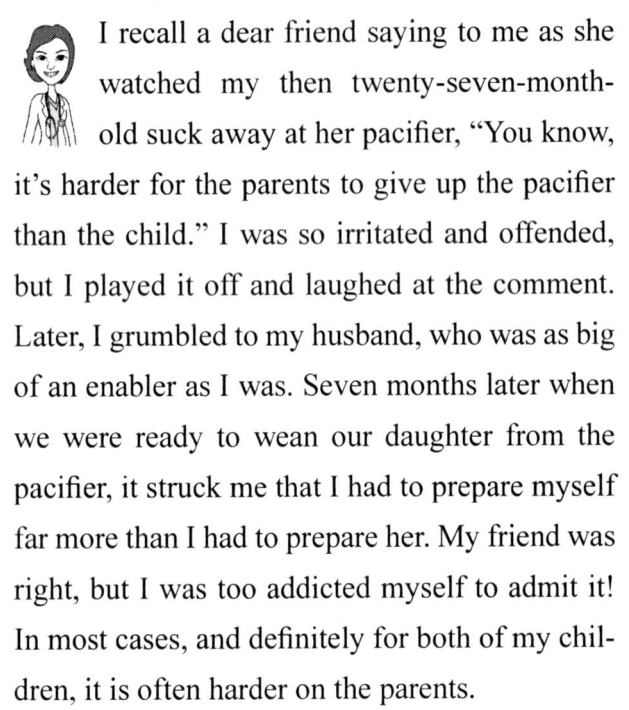

I recall a dear friend saying to me as she watched my then twenty-seven-month-old suck away at her pacifier, "You know, it's harder for the parents to give up the pacifier than the child." I was so irritated and offended, but I played it off and laughed at the comment. Later, I grumbled to my husband, who was as big of an enabler as I was. Seven months later when we were ready to wean our daughter from the pacifier, it struck me that I had to prepare myself far more than I had to prepare her. My friend was right, but I was too addicted myself to admit it! In most cases, and definitely for both of my children, it is often harder on the parents.

Sucking Secret #1:

The pacifier or thumb can soothe the parents just as much as the child and can create a co-dependent habit. Just accept that and move on.

Step 2

Knowledge Is Power: Understanding non-nutritive sucking and soothing

To understand why babies get so hooked on the pacifier or thumb, it is helpful to know why infants love to suck in the first place. Non-nutritive sucking is the natural desire to suck that all babies are born with, which helps them actually latch to a breast or a bottle for nutritive sucking. This sucking reflex or instinct starts well before birth and has been seen on sonogram as early as eighteen weeks of pregnancy, but typical sucking motions are seen around twenty-four weeks. The reflex to suck disappears on its own in the first few months of life, but voluntary sucking will last longer if a habit develops.

Sucking Theories

Somewhere in that first year of life the pacifier and/or thumb transitions from being part of an instinct to an actual intention. There are lots of theories on how sucking becomes a habit, and most of the theories are from the psychology literature and focus on thumb sucking.

Dr. Ruby says:

Although many of these theories may sound archaic or outdated, they are still the foundation for current concepts of child development.

Just an instinct

Dr. Sigmund Freud, the well-known psychiatrist from the early 1900s, believed that thumb sucking was an instinctual activity, or "innate" (something we are born with). He developed a theory of child development that is still accepted by many psychology experts today. He came up with four stages of development, including the oral stage, anal stage, genital stage, and phallic stage. During each stage, a child has certain needs and demands related to the erogenous zones of the mouth, the anus, or the genital region. The first stage of development is the oral stage, which lasts from birth to eighteen months. During this phase of development, the mouth is the primary erogenous zone, meaning infants have a strong desire to suck. All pleasure is directed toward the lips and mouth, which accept food, milk, and other objects. This explains why infants and toddlers love the pacifier, thumb, and whatever else they can put in their eager little mouths. Freud believed that thumb sucking happened when there was a split between the desire to please the erogenous zone (i.e., lips) and the desire to take nourishment.

A bad habit that must be broken
While Freud viewed sucking as innate, the behaviorist John B. Watson rejected instinct as an explanation for this behavior. In *The Psychological Care of Infant and Child* (1928), he proposed that these behaviors resulted from "conditioning" (a learned response). Thumb sucking was just a bad habit that came from a conditioned response

to suck associated with eating that needed to be "cured" within the first few days after birth.

Suck a little longer during feeding

An opposing theory during that time put forward by Dr. David Levy linked the development of thumb sucking with inadequate sucking during feeding. In the first edition of *The Common Sense Book of Baby and Child Care* (1945), Dr. Benjamin Spock recommended increasing the time taken in breast- or bottle-feeding young infants to discourage thumb sucking, but cautioned parents against using restraints such as aluminum mittens, which were used for older children during that era.

Mommy Liza says:

Can you even imagine using aluminum mittens on your child? How times have changed. I can just see the expressions of horror on the faces of the moms in my playgroup if I showed up with aluminum mittens on my son's hands! Needless to say, this is *not* one of our recommended steps!

Mere sport

Charles Anderson Aldrich and Mary Aldrich, the authors of *Babies are Human Beings* (1938), by contrast, viewed thumb sucking as a way to exercise the facial muscles (like a prenatal sport) and suggested that a child would stop this "sport" as soon as he developed other interests.

To Soothe or Not to Soothe…

Whether sucking on the pacifier or thumb is a Freudian urge, a bad habit, a response to not sucking enough during feeds, or mere sport, it is also a method of self-soothing.

Soothing behaviors for a child are similar to stress reducers for an adult. The fact of the matter is that we all need stress reducers in our lives, and we all need ways to sooth ourselves. As adults, we might do yoga or meditate, go for a workout at the gym, have a glass of wine, or pay a visit to our therapist. And at the end of the day, when we need to relax so we can fall asleep, we may watch an entertaining television show, read an interesting book, or spend quality time with our significant other.

Clearly, children don't have these options. Their choices are limited, and what often feels best is sucking. Many parents are comforted by the fact that nearly all babies suck their fingers in the womb and that thumb sucking in infancy is just a natural continuation of this self-soothing behavior. But if you are afraid of a long-lasting habit, then you need to work on alternative stress reducers (discussed in step 11). No one is born with the knowledge of how to do yoga or mediate, so how can we assume a child is born with knowledge of how to soothe without sucking?

Sucking Secret #2:
Despite which non-nutritive sucking theory you agree with, the bottom line is that infants are born with this survival instinct to suck and feed. Because this necessity creates pleasure, it can easily turn into a habit.

Step 3

Making the Decision: Weighing the pros and cons

This book isn't just about making the decision to stop pacifier use or thumb sucking, it's also about the pros and cons of starting in the first place.

For example, a new parent might be concerned about problems with breastfeeding and so-called nipple confusion with the pacifier. There are also fears about the effects on the teeth. And what about that good old stigma of the overindulgent baby sucking her little heart out on the pacifier? Maggie Simpson, look out!

Some Pros
Pain relief
Rest assured, there are plenty of medical benefits for the pacifier too. Pacifiers have long been

used for pain relief and anxiety prevention. The American Academy of Pediatrics (AAP) lists pacifier use as one of the key methods to relieve pain for infants who have undergone emergency room procedures. Most of the studies on infant pain relief have involved using a sugar solution for soothing, but the solution in addition to the pacifier appears to have an even stronger effect. And some studies of newborns showed that using the pacifier was even better than a sugar solution.

Though there are no specific studies on the thumb and pain, it makes sense that the same sucking action on the thumb would provide pain relief.

Dr. Sumi says:

I tried my hardest to limit my girls' pacifier use to sleep time, long car rides, and, well, just bad days. But the exception to that rule was doctor visits, especially at vaccine time. For my patients, I encourage parents to offer the pacifier or breastfeed, if not during the vaccinations, at least immediately afterward.

Feeding premature infants

The pacifier has been shown to help premature infants learn to suck, feed from the bottle, and therefore leave the hospital to go home sooner. Even though the AAP recommends that full-term infants avoid using a pacifier until one month of age, it recommends that premies use a pacifier as soon as they will take it to help them learn to suck.

SIDS prevention

The pacifier's recent claim to fame is its link to reducing occurrences of Sudden Infant Death Syndrome (SIDS). It's not exactly clear how the pacifier reduces SIDS, but researchers think it could be one or more of the following: it might prevent infants from rolling on to their stomachs, it might make them lighter sleepers, it might help the airway stay open, and it could decrease acid reflux and sleep apnea. The AAP recommends that the pacifier be given to babies at night to help prevent SIDS, in addition to putting babies to sleep on their backs. However, the pacifier should never be forced upon an infant, and if he spits it out, it is best not to try putting it back in. So for those parents standing faithfully next to the crib ready to stick the pacifier back in your little one's mouth as soon as it falls out, no need, just go back to bed!

To date, there is no link between thumb sucking and SIDS prevention, but there is no concern that it would increase the risk of SIDS either.

Some Cons

The three biggest areas of concern for pacifier use are that it might interfere with breastfeeding, create dental health problems, and cause infection. The table at the end of this step is a nice summary of all of the pros and cons.

Breastfeeding

Some studies have shown a link between early breast weaning and pacifier use. However, more recent studies have mixed results, with the majority showing no direct link between pacifier use and breastfeeding problems. Some researchers think that enthusiastic pacifier use is more likely a marker of breastfeeding difficulties as opposed to the actual cause of early weaning.

In order to promote breastfeeding, the World Health Organization (WHO) came up with "Baby-friendly Hospital Initiative" in the 1990s, which strongly recommends against the pacifier for breastfeeding babies. The American Academy of Family Physicians (AAFP) recommends that mothers get all the facts about the pros and cons of the pacifier right after birth with assistance from hospital staff to avoid pacifiers if desired. The AAP recommends that the pacifier should not be used when starting to breastfeed and should be postponed until breastfeeding habits are well-established (usually at about one month).

Studies on the thumb and breastfeeding are mixed, but overall they suggest that thumb sucking does not play a big role in breast weaning.

Dental effects
Some good news about the pacifier and dental health is that there is no clear link between cavities and the pacifier, assuming it is not coated with any sweet liquids. The news isn't that great in terms of teeth misalignment (called malocclu-

sions). Some studies have already shown mouth changes like "anterior open bite," "posterior cross bite," and "narrow intercuspid width" occur by three years of age. (*Translation—huge dental bills if the sucking and misalignment continues!*) However, the most significant changes appear to happen if the child continues sucking after age four.

Surprisingly, given all the advertising on various pacifier types, hardly any studies have been done to show that orthodontic pacifiers are better for teeth than the conventional ones. The American Dental Association (ADA) and American Academy of Pediatric Dentistry (AAPD) currently recommend that pacifier use and thumb sucking stop after age four. While both the pacifier and thumb can have bad effects on the teeth, the ADA and AAPD suggest that pacifier use is the better choice from the dental perspective since it's easier to wean a child from the pacifier than the thumb.

Making the Decision

Infections

Cultures have been collected on pacifiers showing that they grow candida (yeast) and bacterial organisms; however, there is no proof that these cultures lead to actual infections or problems in the mouth. A large study including more than 10,000 infants in the United Kingdom looked at pacifier use and thumb sucking at fifteen months of age and their association with infection and health at eighteen months of age. The infants who sucked pacifiers had more earaches and colic than the thumb-sucking group, but it's important to know that the authors could not conclude that the pacifier was the actual cause of any illness.

Studies show that unlimited pacifier use seems to have a stronger association with ear infections (otitis media) than limited use (like for sleep time only). No link between thumb sucking and ear infections has been found. In order to reduce ear infections, the AAFP and AAP recommend that pacifier use be reduced or stopped completely somewhere between six and twelve months of life.

Dr. Sumi says:

In theory, six months is a great time to stop the pacifier, since infants enter a new level of awareness and can be distracted with other objects of affection. In reality, this is also a time period of teething and sleep training when both parents and infants are in a state of "awareness" of how fond they are of the pacifier. So remember, these are guidelines not dogma.

Speech and language

Whether or not the pacifier or thumb causes problems with speech and language is debatable. While earlier studies had conflicting results, a more recent study did show a greater chance of speech disorders in children who sucked their fingers or used a pacifier beyond age three. Long-term use of the pacifier can cause dental problems and contribute to ear infections, which could then lead to speech problems. Some experts say that talking with the pacifier in the mouth not only disrupts speech, but it can also affect position and movement of the tongue with potential to cause a lisp over time. Since long-term thumb sucking can

Making the Decision

lead to the same dental problems as the pacifier, it can theoretically lead to speech problems too.

Thumb deformities
In addition to blisters, sores, and cuts on the thumb, there have been reports of deformities of the bones in thumb suckers that might require surgery for correction. Sometimes the bone changes are just cosmetic, but if they affect a joint, they could affect regular use of the thumb too.

Dr. Sumi's Pacifier Safety Tips:

If you choose to use the pacifier, here are some tips:

1. Be on the lookout for product recalls provided by the U.S. Consumer Product Safety Commission (www.cpsc.gov). The actual pacifier "requirements" can be found at http://www.cpsc.gov/BUSINFO/regsumpacifier.pdf.

Health Effects of the Pacifier and Thumb

Type of Non-Nutritive Sucking	Pros	Cons	What Medical Guidelines Say
Pacifier	• Pain relief • Premature infants learn to suck and feed • SIDS prevention	• Breastfeeding difficulties • Dental effects • Ear infections • Speech effects	• AAP recommends for pain relief up to six months of age • AAP recommends for SIDS prevention after breastfeeding is well-established • AAFP recommends that moms learn about pros/cons with hospital cooperation • AAPD/ADA recommend to stop the pacifier after age four • AAP/AAFP recommend to restrict or stop pacifier after age six months and before age one year to prevent ear infections
Thumb*	• Pain relief (assumed but not proven)	• Dental effects • Speech effects • Thumb deformities	• AAPD/ADA recommend to stop thumb sucking after age four

AAP (American Academy of Pediatrics), AAFP (American Academy of Family Physicians), AAPD (American Academy of Pediatric Dentistry), ADA (American Dental Association)

* Remember, we use the word "thumb" in this book to mean any finger

Making the Decision

2. The safest pacifiers are thought to be silicone and manufactured as only one piece, which means less chance of a part ripping off and causing choking.

3. Latex pacifiers are still made, but they are more likely to be contaminated with fungus and bacteria over time than silicone. The material also breaks down more easily than silicone. The good news is neither silicone nor latex contain the hormone-disrupting chemicals BPA (Bisphenol-A) or phthalates.

4. Never attach strings or ribbons that could choke your baby around the neck or in the mouth.

5. Keep sweets away—don't dip a pacifier into sugar, syrup, or other sweet substances.

6. Keep it clean and replace it if it starts to look worn—wash well with soap and hot water, and make sure the material is dishwasher safe.

Sucking Secret #3:

The main benefits to using the pacifier are pain relief, SIDS prevention, and even thumb-sucking prevention. The main risks are potential effects on breastfeeding if started too early, dental problems, and ear infections. The thumb may help with soothing but can cause dental problems and thumb deformities. Choose your vice and suck wisely!

Making the Decision

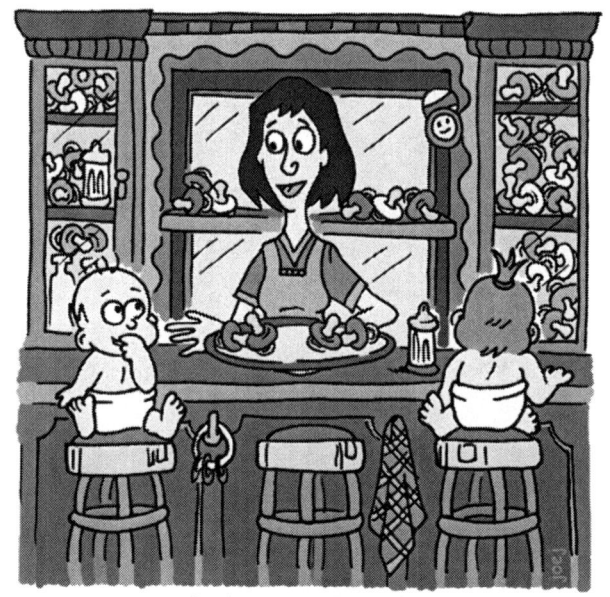

"Silicone or latex?"

Step 4

Appreciating Differences: Cultural perspectives

A Brief History of Pacifying
There's nothing new under the sun. Babies have always cried, toddlers have always thrown tantrums, and parents have always come to the end of their ropes. Throughout history, weary parents have searched for ways to pacify their children—and found that giving their children something to suck on often does the trick.

Dating back to 1000 BC
Over 3,000 years ago, parents in ancient Greece gave their children clay "pacifiers" shaped like animals (horse and frog figures have been discovered by archeologists). In the first century AD, breast-shaped objects made of pottery were given to Roman babies to suck on.

Beginning in the 1500s, babies in northern Europe sucked on small cloth bags filled with various foods. In Europe and Russia these "sugar-tits" or "sugar-rags" contained lumps of meat, bread, or fish. In Finland they contained lumps of animal fat. In Germanic areas, they were called *lutschbeutel* and contained sweetened bread or poppy seeds.

In the 1700s it was fashionable for wealthy British and American parents to give babies sticks of coral to suck on with silver or gold bells attached.

Pacifier fever
As sap from rubber trees began to be used in commercial products, the first pacifier with a rubber nipple was created and patented in 1900. The pacifier hit the bigtime in 1908 when it debuted in the widely read Sears Roebuck catalogue.

As rubber became more refined, more companies started making pacifiers. By 1935, one of the most popular pacifier brands was Binky, from which the pacifier has derived its modern-day nickname.

Appreciating Differences

Pacifier aversion

Foreshadowing its ongoing controversy, the modern-day pacifier's entry into the marketplace was rocky. In 1909, the *New York Times* published an article denouncing the pacifier, calling it a "menace to health," especially among poorer classes.

Though popular in Britain, the pacifier was seen as unsanitary and condemned by many healthcare professionals in the early twentieth century. It was pronounced a "perverted American ingenuity" and a "curse of babyhood." "Remember," one author warned of the pacifier's addictive qualities, "that a baby that has had a dummy [the British term for pacifier] is like a tiger that has tasted blood." In 1926, similar disdain in France led to a national ban on the sale of the pacifier, or *sucette*.

Mommy Liza says:

Today the pacifier isn't so harshly criticized thanks to a better understanding of sanitation…although I've spotted kids sucking on some pretty unsanitary pacifiers! I've seen parents use the "five-second rule" when a pacifier falls on a public floor or "wash off" the pacifier in their own mouths before giving it back to their kids. Parents, these are no-nos. Always pack a spare in the diaper bag or thoroughly wash a pacifier with soap and warm water when it falls on the floor.

Cultural Differences

In Western societies, an estimated 75 to 90 percent of newborns are pacifier or thumb suckers. Studies show that a significant number of these infants prolong their sucking habits well into childhood.

Mommy Liza says:

With my background in social history and cultural disparities, I wanted to take a look at how sucking habits differ between countries and cultures. My friends from different cultures shared their own observations with me too. My British friend says that pacifiers are a little taboo in Britain. Although British parents may want to give their child a pacifier, often they don't for fear they'll be criticized. An Italian friend told me that pacifiers are not really looked down upon in Italy as long as a child gives it up by age three. When a child doesn't self-wean, the parents just throw the pacifier out and endure a few rough days while the child goes "cold turkey."

Some interesting trends

Sucking habits are much more prominent in industrialized countries (like the United States, where pacifier use among infants has been estimated as high as 74 percent) than in developing countries (like Africa, where one researcher claims that sucking rates are so universally low that they're not worth researching). This may be because developing countries have much higher rates of breastfeeding. In developing countries, 38 percent of infants are exclusively breastfed (i.e., receive only breastmilk, no formula) for the first six months of life, compared to the United States where less than 14 percent of infants are exclusively breastfed for the same period of time.

Rates in industrialized countries

Rates of pacifier use in the United States are some

of the highest in the world, and U.S. children tend to continue the habit until they are much older. One study in the States showed that over 20 percent of children have a sucking habit until age three or older. Interestingly, the mothers in this study were more likely to be older and have a higher education level, while other studies have shown higher pacifier rates in children of mothers who were younger with lower education levels.

The United States is not the only country that lets their children suck and suck and suck. Non-nutritive sucking habits have also been observed to be prevalent among children in other industrialized nations. In the United Kingdom, roughly 66 percent of zero to six-month-olds use pacifiers and more than 57 percent of fifteen-month-olds suck a pacifier or thumb. Studies in Sweden show that 87 percent of babies ages two to eighteen months are pacifier or thumb suckers. In Western Australia, 66 percent of three-month-olds use pacifiers.

Rates in developing countries
Developing countries are very different. Both

pacifier use and finger sucking are far less common, and most children do not display a desire to suck once weaned from the breast (*must be nice*). A study in rural Zimbabwe showed that only 2 percent of infants ages zero to two years are pacifier or digit suckers. Similarly, in rural areas of India, children do not display a desire for nonnutritive sucking. In New Zealand, pacifier use at fifteen weeks was 5 percent in the more rural South Island and 32 percent in the more urban North Island. Studies conducted in American Indian tribes found that almost no infants engage in pacifier or digit sucking.

So why all of the differences?
Reasons that these children may not have the "paci urge" are thought to be related to breastfeeding. Often babies in rural areas or developing regions are breastfed and allowed to suck at their mothers' breasts to their hearts' desire. Decreased milk production, due to the mother's poor nourishment or hard labor during the day, causes the child to have to suck longer in order to receive enough milk, which probably fulfills her

innate desire to suck.

We put together a table to show rates of breastfeeding and pacifier use in industrialized versus developing countries. Most of the information shown in the table is from the World Health Organization. You'll notice that rates of breastfeeding are highest while rates of pacifier use are lowest in developing countries as compared to industrialized countries. Unfortunately, we weren't able to find many studies documenting the rates of thumb sucking, so that information wasn't included.

Sucking Secret #4:
Parents have been pacifying their babies for thousands of years with a variety of different objects. The popularity of the pacifier has had its ups and downs, and there are definitely cultural trends. Urban societies use the pacifier and thumb more than their rural counterparts who typically breastfeed more. This could be a case of the artificial versus human pacifier.

Health Effects of the Pacifier and Thumb

Region/Country	Exclusive Breastfeeding Rate	Prevalence of Non-Nutritive Sucking (Pacifier)
Developing Countries	six months: 38 percent	Not available
Industrialized Countries	Not available	75–90 percent
Africa	six months: Western and Southern regions 54 to 88 percent Northern regions 28 percent	Not available
Central America	three months: 40 percent	Not available
Central and Eastern Europe/ the Commonwealth of Independent States	six months: 19 percent	Not available
East Asia/ Pacific	six months: 43 percent	Not available
Egypt	six months: 53 percent	20 percent
Finland	five months: 3 percent	75 percent
India	six months: 46 percent	Not available
Italy	six months: 5 percent	73 percent
Japan	six months: 21 percent	12.5 percent
South America	three months: 38 percent	Not available
South Asia	six months: 45 percent	Not available
United Kingdom	six months: 10 percent	42 percent
United States	six months: 13.6 percent	74 percent

Step 5

Turning to Others: A survey of what parents think

While we have a lot of personal and professional experience to offer you, sometimes it helps to get information straight from the horse's mouth. So we decided to conduct a survey of our patients, parenting discussion groups, family, and friends. We asked what they thought about pacifier and thumb sucking and what worked/didn't work as far as weaning goes.

We had over 100 parents respond to our surveys, and we found out some surprising information. Almost every parent who responded said his or her child used the pacifier or thumb. Most parents reported beginning to use the pacifier or encouraging thumb sucking because it was a good way to stop the baby from crying. One parent even admitted it was due to "pure laziness," but the majority felt like it was "preservation of sanity."

Pacifier Survey Results

Age pacifier use started

We also found that the majority of babies (73 percent) started to use the pacifier within the first month of life. Some even began at the hospital. For those who started at the hospital, it was usually given by the nurses, especially for infants in the intensive care unit.

Age Pacifier Use Began

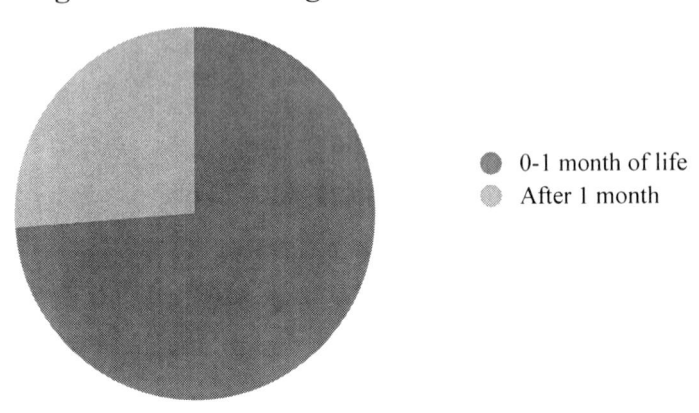

- 0-1 month of life
- After 1 month

Many of the parents we sampled also breastfed, which contradicts the theory that newborns who use the pacifier develop nipple confusion and have trouble breastfeeding. Granted our sample size was small and is clearly not representative of every person in the entire country. Also, if you refer back to step 3, you'll see that medical organizations are still cautious about recommending the pacifier until the baby can latch and breastfeed well.

Age at pacifier weaning

In our sample, weaning took place at various ages, ranging from three months to over three years of age. The majority weaned between one and three years of age. The method parents used also varied from cold turkey, to bribery, to a fairy, to losing it.

Age Pacifier Use Ended

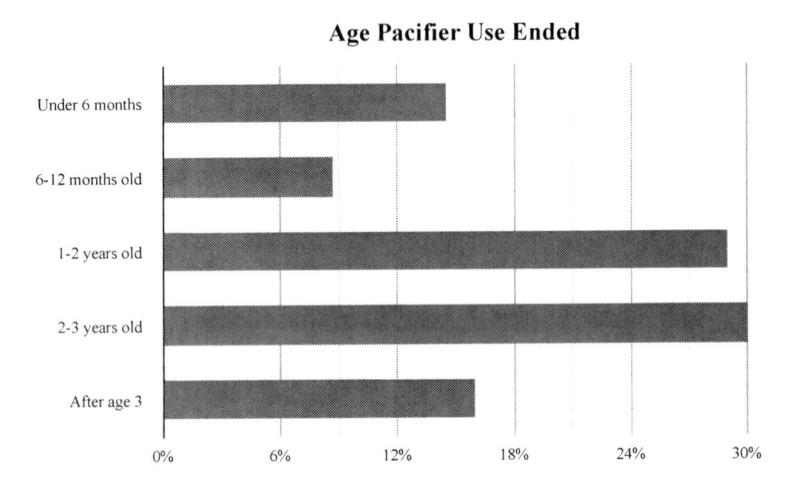

Age	Percentage
Under 6 months	~15%
6-12 months old	~9%
1-2 years old	~28%
2-3 years old	~30%
After age 3	~16%

How long it took to wean

As far as the length of time it took, it ranged from one day to longer than one month with multiple relapses. The cold-turkey method was the most popular weaning method.

Dr. Sumi says:

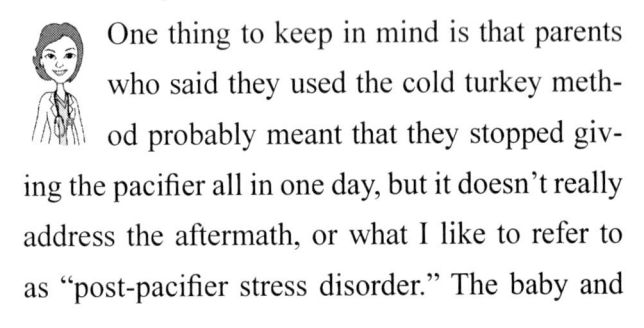

One thing to keep in mind is that parents who said they used the cold turkey method probably meant that they stopped giving the pacifier all in one day, but it doesn't really address the aftermath, or what I like to refer to as "post-pacifier stress disorder." The baby and parents are both victims of this period of fussiness, whining, and sleepless nights! Typically, this lasts a week with a hint of relapse here and there afterward.

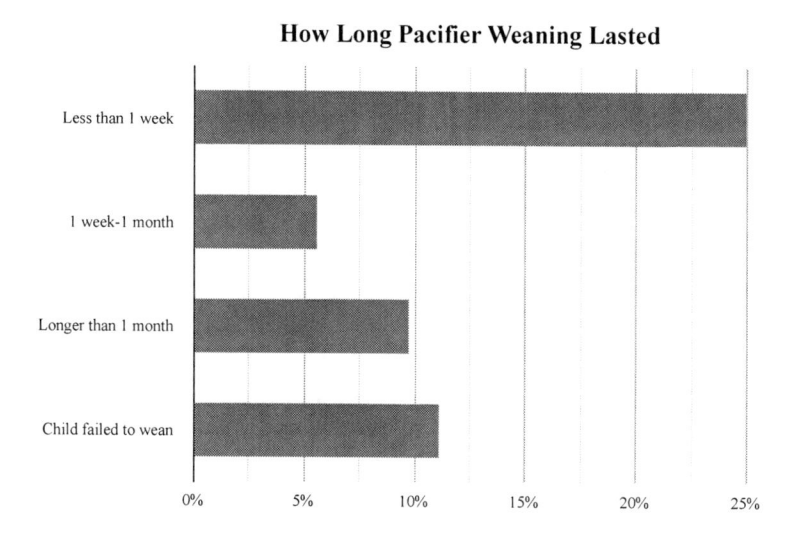

How Long Pacifier Weaning Lasted

Category	Percentage
Less than 1 week	~25%
1 week-1 month	~6%
Longer than 1 month	~10%
Child failed to wean	~12%

Ear infections and dental problems
Use of the pacifier did not seem to be related to ear infections, despite research suggesting that it is. However, this may be due to the fact that most of our respondents were parents who also breastfed their children, and breastfeeding is linked to fewer cases of ear infections. Also, only a few

parents (less than 10 percent) reported that their children had dental problems as a result of using the pacifier, probably because most children were weaned by age three.

Thumb Sucking Survey

Age thumb sucking started

Our research on thumb suckers was similar in most respects, but we did find some surprising results. For example, most parents reported that thumb sucking started later. However, that is not the case for all children. One parent reported that the baby sucked in utero and was born with a "sucking-blister" on his wrist, but could not reliably get his thumb in his mouth until three months old.

Mommy Liza says:

In my daily experience, pacifier users far outnumber thumb suckers. Like our study has found, I've noticed that most pacifier users start the habit in the first few weeks of life while most thumb suckers begin much later. I know several children who rejected the pacifier as newborns but then became avid thumb suckers out of the blue when they were seven to ten months old.

Age Thumb Use Began

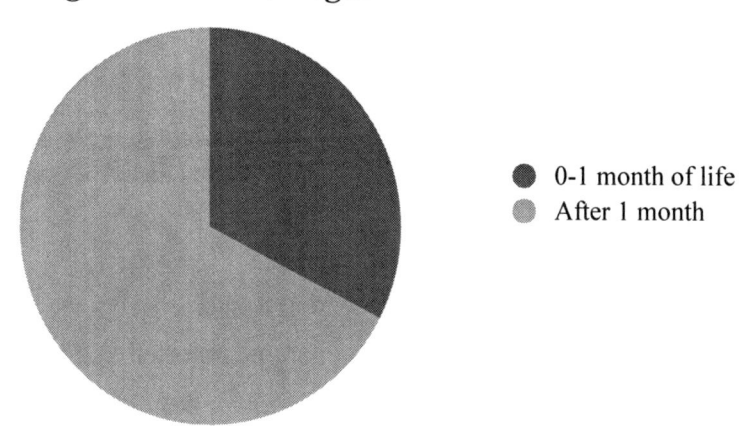

- 0-1 month of life
- After 1 month

Age thumb sucking stopped

Most of the respondents also reported that weaning happens at a much later age (about 75 percent reported their child weaned after age three). One parent even reported that her child is nine years old and is still sucking his thumb.

Age Thumb Use Ended

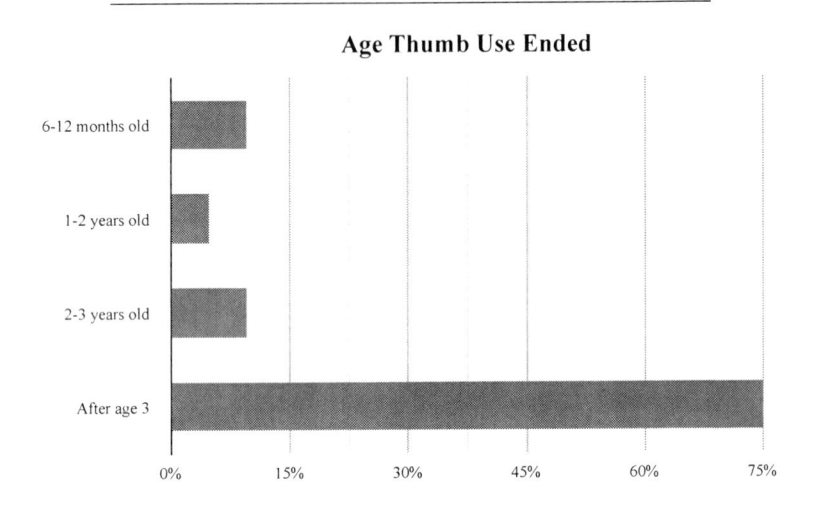

Age	Percentage
6-12 months old	~8%
1-2 years old	~3%
2-3 years old	~8%
After age 3	~75%

Weaning methods and how long it took

The good news is that most parents reported that even though the process was gradual, their child self-weaned. For those who did not self-wean, parents used a finger guard of some sort, such as tape or a Band-Aid or a finger guard you can purchase. Other children stopped on their own after the dentist told them it would cause teeth deformities. It is interesting to note that many babies developed the thumb habit only after giving up the pacifier.

Turning to Others

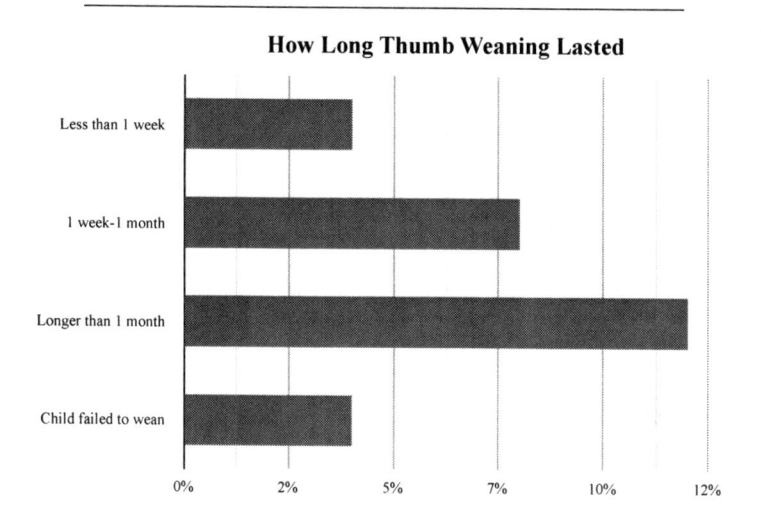

How Long Thumb Weaning Lasted

Category	Percentage
Less than 1 week	~3%
1 week-1 month	~7%
Longer than 1 month	~11%
Child failed to wean	~3%

Ear infections and dental problems

Similar to the pacifier survey results, not many parents reported that their children had an increase in episodes of ear infections or dental problems as a result of thumb sucking. Since most of these kids sucked their thumbs after age three, the lack of dental problems is a little surprising.

Sucking Secret #5:

Pacifier use tends to start earlier but also ends earlier. Thumb use starts later but ends later. Many different weaning techniques can be used for pacifier suckers, with cold turkey being the most common, while thumb sucking usually stops naturally.

Step 6

Getting Ready for the Big Day: Deciding when to make a clean break

From a psychological and child development perspective, most children are ready to give up the pacifier when they are between twelve and eighteen months old.

The World According to Freud
According to Freud, there are four stages of child development (see step 2), and if you sail through those stages, you become a "well-developed" adult. After eighteen months of age, a child moves on from the oral stage and progresses on to the anal stage. During this stage of development, a child's erogenous zone becomes the anus, with a

focus on stooling or holding it in. Therefore, this stage is an ideal time for the child to move away from the pacifier and to focus on potty training. Also, Freud goes on to say that if children do not "resolve" each stage successfully, than an entire slew of problems can arise. For example, a child can become orally fixated, meaning they never outgrow the need to suck. These are the people who later become overeaters, smokers, etc. Of course this view doesn't fully explain these behaviors, and there are no studies to link these behaviors to pacifier or thumb use, but if you want to read more about Freud's theory, refer to the resource section in the back of the book.

Dr. Sumi says:

If you feel like you are reading some contradictory information in this book, it's only because the science is far from perfect. Medical guidelines typically say wean under age one, while dental guidelines say to do so by age four. Now the psychologists are giving us yet a different age. So what's the right answer? I'm sorry to say, my friend, it is somewhere after six months and before age four! However, as you read more, we'll give you the tools to help narrow that range down for yourself.

What Happens in Real Life

Now that we know what Freud thought, let's talk about what happens in real life. It's great to know that, in theory, your child should wean by eighteen months, but it's not that easy. Some children just aren't ready to wean at that age. What Freud's theory assumes is that every child is the same, but we all know that isn't the case. We are firm believers that you need to understand your child's temperament, behaviors, and reasons for using the thumb/pacifier so that you know the best approach to take for weaning and when to take it!

- In preparing for the big day, we suggest first determining whether the sucking is an emotional habit or an empty one. An "emotional habit" has a cause or reason behind it, usually due to stress in the environment that can then serve as a trigger. An "empty habit" has no underlying cause. Stressors in the environment that may cause the habit or make it worse include things like moving to a new house or birth of a new sibling. If there is no evidence of stress, the sucking may be an empty habit.

- If the sucking is an empty habit, then you should be able to use a simplified approach, such as praising children for not sucking, rather than punishing or yelling when they do suck. In psychological terms, this approach of praising the child is called positive reinforcement. The idea is that you ignore the bad behavior and praise the good behavior, which leads to more good behavior (i.e., not sucking).

Dr. Ruby says:

This positive approach is great for all types of undesirable behaviors (e.g., following directions, hitting, throwing toys) not just pacifier/thumb sucking. Sometimes I tell the parents to "catch 'em being GOOD." You can even set a timer and every time the timer goes off you can look to see if the child is sucking. If the child is not sucking, then shower him with praise.

Getting Ready for the Big Day

If he is, then you just ignore the behavior.

- If a child is sucking because of boredom, be creative and come up with an activity.

Dr. Ruby says:

I always revert to reading books when my child gets bored. Why not cure boredom and boost vocabulary at the same time!

- If the child is older, you can ask her what would make it easier to stop sucking, or if there is something else she would rather do.
- You can even bring your child to the dentist to "encourage" her to stop sucking by telling her what could happen to her teeth if she does not stop sucking.
- If sucking is an emotional habit and has a cause or is linked to a stressor, then try to address the stressor and remove it if possible. We as parents often take on too much and think we can do everything; however, it's okay to ask for help. Your doctor may

be able to help you figure out or lessen the stressor, or you can take your child to a therapist. For example, if the child has just started using the pacifier or is now refusing to give it up, look for reasons why this may be happening. Think of yourself as a detective. Try to figure out what has changed in the environment (if anything). As a child psychologist, here are some questions I would ask:

Getting Ready for the Big Day

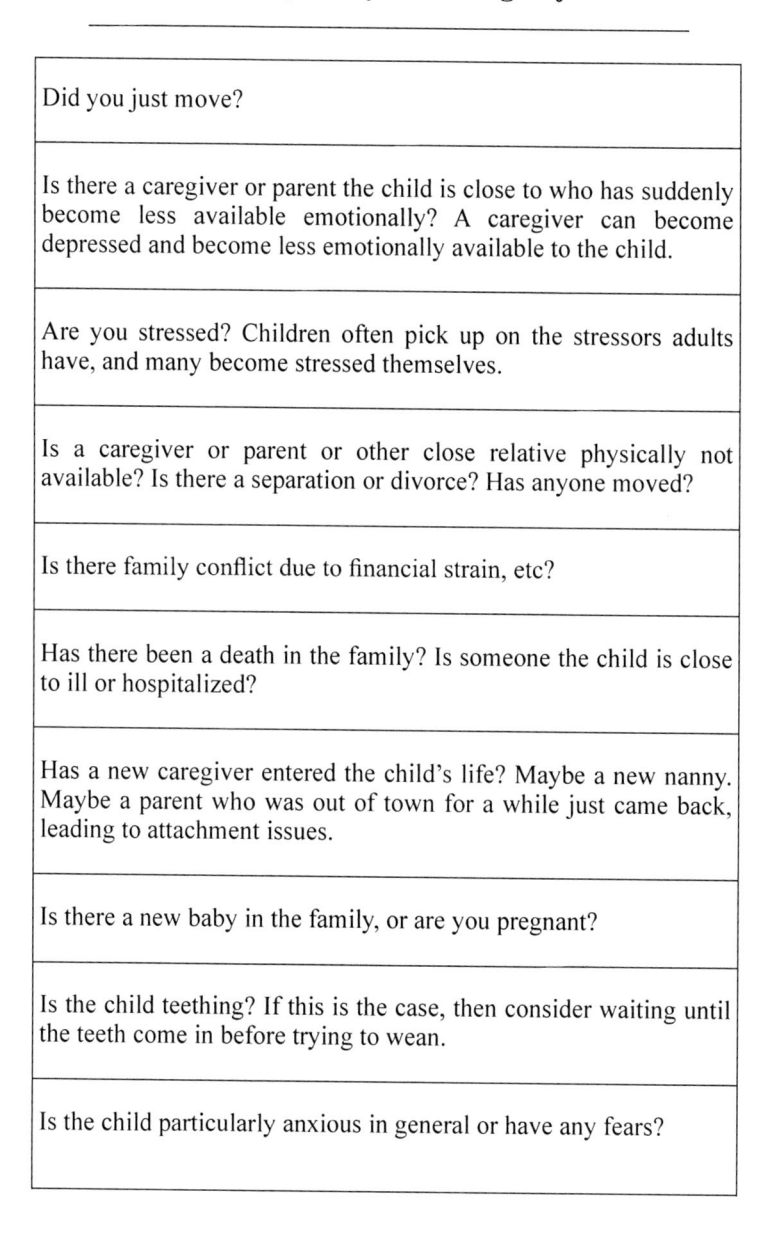

Did you just move?
Is there a caregiver or parent the child is close to who has suddenly become less available emotionally? A caregiver can become depressed and become less emotionally available to the child.
Are you stressed? Children often pick up on the stressors adults have, and many become stressed themselves.
Is a caregiver or parent or other close relative physically not available? Is there a separation or divorce? Has anyone moved?
Is there family conflict due to financial strain, etc?
Has there been a death in the family? Is someone the child is close to ill or hospitalized?
Has a new caregiver entered the child's life? Maybe a new nanny. Maybe a parent who was out of town for a while just came back, leading to attachment issues.
Is there a new baby in the family, or are you pregnant?
Is the child teething? If this is the case, then consider waiting until the teeth come in before trying to wean.
Is the child particularly anxious in general or have any fears?

Dr. Ruby says:

Before you go jumping to conclusions, ask any other caregivers who are close to the child to confirm or dispel your belief.

- If a child is sucking when feeling anxious or needing comfort, focus instead on correcting the cause of the anxiety and provide comfort to your child. For example, a child may be uncomfortable around the household dog or cat, so she may begin sucking every time the pet enters the room. You have two options: get rid of the pet or teach your child an alternate coping mechanism to sucking to deal with the anxiety.
- If there is an identifiable cause to the sucking (or inability to wean) that you feel is beyond your capabilities, then a therapist can work with the child to help him cope with some of these issues. For example, grief therapy is very effective in dealing with loss. Dyadic therapy (one-on-one parent-child therapy) is great for

Getting Ready for the Big Day

attachment issues. Play therapy is great for family conflict. A seasoned therapist can easily address these issues with you and your child, so don't be afraid or embarrassed to seek help.

Sucking Secret #6:

Determine what motivates your little one to suck and assess any stressors in the environment. Know your limits. If you are having an extremely difficult time with weaning, or if you think it may be related to something else going on in your life, you can always ask for help.

Step 7

Making a List: What weaning techniques have other parents used?

Believe it or not, there are countless methods for weaning that can be found just about anywhere including reference books, magazines, advice from friends, family, and sometimes nosy strangers, and of course the almighty Internet. We narrowed down a long list of weaning methods to twelve widely used and successful techniques.

#1 Cold-Turkey approach: This speaks for itself. You basically take the pacifier from the child and endure blood-curdling screaming until the child gets used to not having one. Well, that's not completely true. Some kids do very well with this approach, and once the pacifier is taken away, they don't seem to mind. It's a common trick for parents to "lose" the pacifier on a trip; many kids just never ask for it again.

Dr. Ruby says:

My grandmother said she pretended to throw my aunt's pacifier out the window as they drove past a farm and said a cow got it. Lucky cow! Beware though, since this approach can sometimes lead to replacing-one-addiction-with-another syndrome. For example, the child gives up the pacifier and switches to the thumb.

#2 Dangle-the-Carrot approach: This approach basically equates to bribery. You offer the child anything and everything to stop using the pacifier or sucking the thumb. It goes something like this: "Sweetie if you give Mommy the binky, I'll let you have a cookie after dinner." One parent who responded to our survey had the child purchase a gift at a toy store in exchange for her collection of pacifiers.

#3 Downsizing or Loss-of-Suck-Appeal approach: Some parents cut a hole in the pacifier so when the child sucks on it, she no longer gets much pleasure from it. The idea behind this method is that the child will no longer want to use the pacifier if it is no longer fulfilling her desire to suck. Some even trim it down over time until there is just nothing left to suck. Be careful with this trick though, since you could be creating a choking hazard if parts break off.

#4 Hit-the-Jackpot approach: The child just self-weans…as if we could all be this lucky. In most cases, self-weaning is probably due to the fact that the child just lost interest at a young age and found other ways to soothe, or the parents inadvertently taught the child other ways to soothe (e.g., hug a stuffed animal, squeeze a blankie, use a rocking chair). This is sometimes the only option for parents of thumb suckers.

#5 Laid-back approach: You may have heard parents say, "The pacifier is not something you should waste time worrying about. You'll find that you have to choose your battles in parenthood if you're gonna remain sane." And, "Talk to parents with autistic children, or children with leukemia, or kids who've been hurt, and they'll tell you what's really worth worrying about." One favorite saying is, "Do you see any kids in college sucking their thumbs? It'll take care of itself way before then!"

#6 Magical-Mythical-Fairy approach: This is similar to the Tooth Fairy. A child looses a tooth and puts it under her pillow, and when she wakes up she finds money instead of the tooth. Some parents have now cleverly created the "Pacifier Fairy" (or some other type of fairy or elf). The story goes…while the child is sleeping, the pacifier fairy flies in and swoops down and takes the pacifier during the night and replaces it with a wonderful gift (a doll or toy, etc).

Dr. Sumi says:

I read a story about the Easter Bunny taking it, and ended up creating the "Good Witch" to help my youngest beat the pacifier at Halloween. The Good Witch brought lots of candy and toys that night in exchange for the prized pacifier. In our survey, parents described a ghost taking it and even a raccoon. There is nothing wrong with using your creativity!

#7 Methodical approach: Some parents are very particular regarding when they will allow their child to begin using the pacifier, at what times during the day or night they can use it, and at what age to stop. It probably doesn't hurt to have a plan in mind, but remember, when dealing with a child, things don't always go as planned. However, there is a sensible gradual way to create a sucking plan for the pacifier or thumb: start by telling your child that it is time to stop using it, except at home, and that soon he won't need it at all. A week or so later, tell him only to use it at bedtime. After that, tell him that he is a big boy and doesn't need it at all. When you're done, throw all the pacifiers away. Too bad you can't throw away the thumb! But you can give your child a special stuffed toy to take to bed to replace the comfort of the thumb or as a reward for not thumb sucking. Keep in mind that the process can take much longer for thumb lovers.

#8 Potions-and-Lotions approach: Parents will put all sorts of things on their kid's pacifier or thumb to make it taste unappealing. Some parents cover the thumb or the hand at night as a reminder to not suck, using bandages, socks, gloves, ace wraps, or anything else that will stay on. You can even purchase specific devices to cover the thumb, which serve as reminders for older children. A more drastic approach for thumb suckers (as a last resort only) are dental appliances placed on the palate, which serve as a painful reminder not to suck!

Dr. Ruby says:

I know my parents would dip my thumb in a "special medicine" the doctor gave them designed to make my thumb taste bad. However, that didn't work well given that I still refused to give it up at the age of four. I read that one parent put fish sauce on the pacifier to make it less appealing. My parents decided to cover my

Making a List

thumb instead.

#9 Rationalization approach (which usually leads to one of the other approaches): Often parents find it extremely difficult to give up the pacifier and then find some key reasons to convince themselves (and other parents and caretakers they might guilt along the way) that "for the good of their child," they must go through with it. You might hear things like, "It's best for my son to learn other ways of falling asleep and self-soothing rather than relying on the pacifier." Or, "Getting rid of the pacifier will help my daughter gain some independence. A few sleepless nights is worth the bigger purpose of helping her become a healthier and happier child."

Dr. Sumi says:

This approach is truly just for parents. First parents have to wean themselves off the idea of the pacifier by rationalizing, and then they can muster the energy to wean their children.

#10 Saying Good-bye: Some parents allow the child to say good-bye and send the pacifier off on its way. For example, they tie it to a balloon and watch it float away.

#11 Unplug-and-Hug approach: You can gently remove the pacifier/thumb from the child's mouth, provide immediate emotional support in the form of a hug or praise, and then proceed to distract the child with another activity.

#12 You're-All-Grown-Up approach: Some parents simply explain to their child that he is becoming a "big boy" now and doesn't need the pacifier anymore. Some even link it to the transition of sleeping in the "big boy" bed. Amazingly, this tactic does work but is most suited for older children who have the vocabulary to understand. Parents can take this a step further and appeal to their child's generous side by asking him to donate the pacifier to a new baby or a child in need or to the doctor to use for another patient. Positive reinforcement with stickers, a chart with a reward at the end of the week, or even small daily

Making a List

rewards are helpful with this approach and all the others too.

Sucking Secret #7:

There are many great techniques for weaning, but don't be afraid to be creative and make up your own version. You can even use a few approaches together.

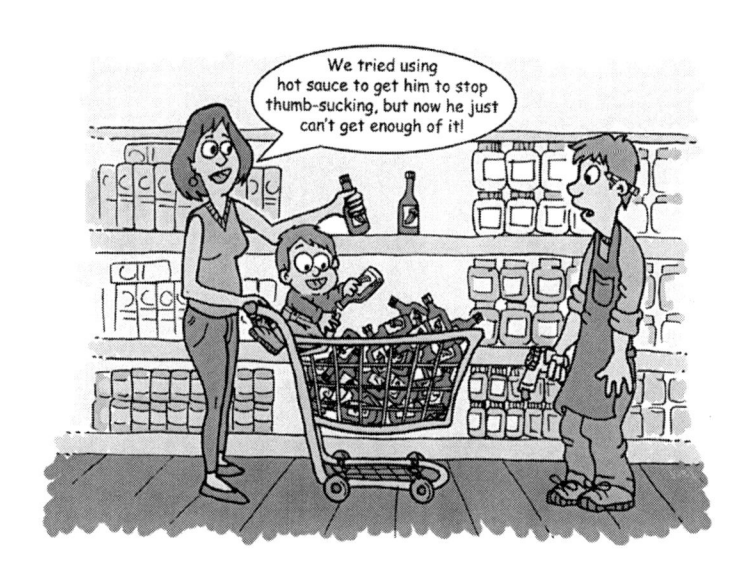

Step 8

Choosing the Technique and Timing: What's best for you and your child

When choosing which weaning approach to use, remember that there is no perfect technique. It's all about what works for you and your child. If you're eager to get the pacifier out of your life, then it makes sense to use the tried-and-true cold-turkey method or something similar to the saying-goodbye technique. If you would rather take it more slowly, no worries, slow and steady is also a good way to be consistent and successful with weaning. For example, when it comes to sleep training, some parents take a more gradual approach. They either don't believe in letting their babies cry at all or they prefer to let them cry for shorter intervals over a longer time period as opposed to the just-let-them-cry-it-all-out method. These parents will probably feel more comfortable with the downsizing, methodological, or unplug-and-hug approaches, which are more gradual.

Dr. Sumi says:

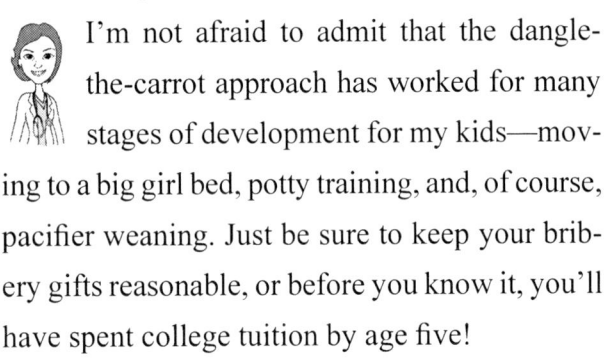

I'm not afraid to admit that the dangle-the-carrot approach has worked for many stages of development for my kids—moving to a big girl bed, potty training, and, of course, pacifier weaning. Just be sure to keep your bribery gifts reasonable, or before you know it, you'll have spent college tuition by age five!

The three Ps:
be Practical, be Positive, avoid Power struggles
While there is no wrong technique, be sure to pick the one that best fits your parenting style so that you can be consistent and follow through. Also be realistic and practical about the timing. For example, if you think your child is not ready because of a new baby in the family or a recent

Choosing the Technique and Timing

move or a new teacher at school, then wait until both you and your child can focus on being consistent with the task. Along those lines, never punish the child for struggling. Be positive and encouraging and understanding. How would you feel if you were giving up eating chocolate and someone yelled at you every time you faltered? It is important to be understanding, especially with older children who have become more addicted to the pacifier or thumb and may take longer to wean and require more preparation. Also, negative reinforcement can be tricky and translate into attention-seeking behavior. You might find your child sucking the pacifier or thumb even more just to get a rise out of you. If weaning is not handled properly, the child's attachment to the item may become a major issue and the source of continuous power struggles. This is not simply unpleasant, it is also unproductive as it generates considerably more stress for everyone.

Dr. Ruby says:

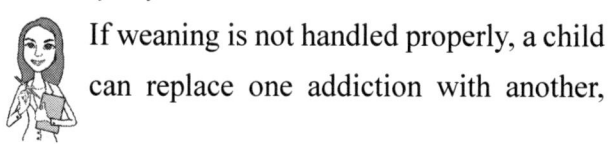

If weaning is not handled properly, a child can replace one addiction with another, and usually the second addiction is actually harder to break. For example, when the pacifier is abruptly taken, the child may switch to the thumb. Why does this happen? Well, it could happen if the child had an emotional sucking habit instead of an empty one, and continues to have a need to self-soothe. In our research, we found that children who suck their thumbs actually suck for more time during the day than pacifier users and have an even harder time giving it up.

Developmental Phases to Consider

Some kids go on to continue sucking the thumb until they are six or seven. Why do they suddenly stop at this age? At this age, peer pressure starts to kick in and kids become too embarrassed to suck because they are teased by their peers. Prior to that age, preschoolers are pretty oblivious to the opinions of their peers. This is a well-known egocentric phase of development in psychology and was first recognized by Jean Piaget. As they emerge from this period, things change, and they become aware of and sensitive to what other kids are thinking and saying about them. Therefore,

Choosing the Technique and Timing

at this point, attachment to their thumbs may no longer be quite so attractive, since it causes more stress than it reduces. Consequently, they become considerably more inspired and inclined to seek out other more socially acceptable alternatives. This is a perfect time to try the you're-all-grown-up approach.

Just remember, if weaning is too abrupt or inconsistent before your child reaches the egocentric phase, she may keep sucking on the pacifier, or replace her addiction with another. This is because she was not able to come up with a better self-soothing strategy, so she reverted back to sucking. This act of reverting to an infantile state rather than moving on is called regression by psychologists.

So, if you're thinking about using the cold-turkey method, it's still a good idea. You're just much better off if you teach your child another self-soothing strategy to replace it, or you could face relapse or replacing the addiction with another habit. We discuss alternate self-soothing strategies in step 11.

Sucking Secret #8:

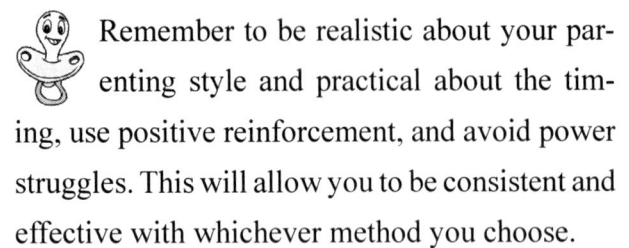

Remember to be realistic about your parenting style and practical about the timing, use positive reinforcement, and avoid power struggles. This will allow you to be consistent and effective with whichever method you choose.

Step 9

Getting the Sponsors On Board: A united front

When an adult commits to breaking a habit, support from others can be critical. It's said that "sponsors" (people designated to support and encourage through times of temptation) are the backbone of quitting programs. Children are no different. They too need people to coach them through behavioral changes. Think of everyone who has responsibility for your child as his sponsor—that's you, your partner, family members, childcare providers, babysitters, church nursery workers, or any other caregivers.

You can avoid frustrations (and the risk of relapse) by making sure your child's caregivers are a united front, and that your child receives only consistent messages. When you'll be away from your child, take action so that each sponsor is as resolute and prepared as you are to help your child kick his habit.

- **Talk amongst yourselves**: Have a serious talk with each of your child's sponsors (starting with your partner, making sure he or she is *completely* on board). Let each person know how important this is for your child and how serious you are about helping her to wean from the pacifier or thumb. Explain the details of your weaning strategy and how essential their role is in your child's success.
- **Share the wealth**: In case your little paddict goes through paci-withdrawal while in their care, arm each sponsor with the wealth of strategies you use in moments of weakness. Share any special activities they can do to distract your child or any soothing techniques (see step 11) that will help them get through those inevitable

Getting the Sponsors On Board

rough spots.

- **It's all about consistency**: Your sponsors should use the same words, tone, and approach with your child as you do. Tell your sponsors exactly what you say to your child when he asks for the paci or starts sucking his thumb and ask them to do the same. Share what you do in the case of a meltdown and how you praise him for a job well done.

- **Secret weapons**: Pack a special bag to drop off with your child's sponsor, filled with "secret weapons" to use if things get rough. These could include a treasured book, a favorite DVD, or even a surprise new toy that your sponsor can give as a reward.

- **The written word**: If a sponsor will be caring for your child overnight, write down your rules and strategies and go over them in detail with the sponsor. Since bedtime can often be hardest for your child, instructions that your sponsor can use for reference will help ensure an overnight stay is a success.

- **The weakest link**: You know who they are. The doting grandparent whose worst nightmare is saying "no" to your child. Or the adoring daddy who's putty in the hands of his little girl. Prepare to pay special attention to those sponsors who tend to give in at the first whimper. If done correctly and with consistency, the weaning process is brief (it typically takes just a week!), so go the extra mile to ensure those "weakest link" sponsors stay strong. You might instruct a grandparent to call you if things become too difficult so you can coach your child through a rough spot (i.e., be the "bad guy," so they don't have to). If you imagine your spouse might cave under pressure, clear your calendar and stay at home during the weaning process so he or she is not tempted to give in while you're away.
- **Praises all around**: When you pick your child up from a sponsor, don't just make a big deal to your child about his success.

Getting the Sponsors On Board

Praise that sponsor too! With sincere interest, ask the sponsor to tell you all about the day and to share any struggles. Truly sympathize with her if she's had a rough time, and praise her to the hilt for a job well done. She'll keep up the good work next time!

Mommy Liza says:

For weeks my friend Heather worked to gradually wean her son from the paci. He was down to the last step: only at bedtime. When she took him to spend the weekend with his grandparents, she told them the rule. To Heather's dismay, her son came home—paci in mouth—with a slew of pictures from the weekend, all showing him sucking away. Because Heather hadn't had a serious talk with her parents, they didn't understand how serious her weaning efforts had been. As a result, they didn't see it as a big deal to give him the pacifier here and there until, before they knew it, he was sucking all the time. Though eventually successful, Heather had to start the weaning process over from scratch due to the setbacks from that weekend.

Sucking Secret #9:

It is important to get the other sponsors/caregivers on board and make sure that everyone in the child's environment is doing the same thing.

Step 10

Turning Fear into Hope: Success stories

Others have been down this road before you and they have success stories to share. These stories come from our patients, the parents we surveyed, and online parenting forums like dcurbanmom.com. Read and smile!

#1 The Pig Ate It
"We were afraid of becoming the bad guys who took the paci away, and we were looking for someone or something else to take the heat! We took our baby to the fair at twenty months. While admiring the pigs, it fell. So that was the end of that. She didn't ask for it much, but our answer was always, 'Sorry dear, the pig ate it.'"

#2 Trash Mouth

"I remember when I was almost four, I put my pacifier in the trash can when a friend came over for a playdate so she wouldn't think I was a baby. My mom conveniently emptied the trash while we played, so there was no going back. It was a scary feeling, but I got over it within a day or so. I'm planning on taking the same 'throw it out' approach for my son, since it worked for me."

#3 Bugs Bunny to the Rescue

"I was so worried about my five-year-old son's thumb sucking. His dad and I had talked to him about cutting back, but we didn't want to give him a complex. One day we were watching a cartoon together and one of the characters had buckteeth. Luckily he asked why the character looked like that, and I explained that it was from sucking on his thumb. He had a scared look on his face and then asked if he would look like that too. I told him that if he stopped now, then he wouldn't. He stopped cold turkey and has never done it again."

#4 Incredible Shrinking Pacifier

"I slowly cut the tips off of my daughter's favorite pacifiers little by little. My eleven-month-old just stopped liking them, and then I just made them disappear."

#5 The Sooner the Better

"I am another mom who believes you should just take the paci away, but I also believe it should be done as early as possible. My daughter loved her paci from day one, but on the advice of a pediatric nurse, we decided we would take it away before she got old enough to really understand and rationalize with us on it. Her advice was to quit between six and nine months. It worked, and I would say that it is probably much easier to take it away slowly or cold turkey when they can't really ask for it."

#6 Selective Sucking

"Weaning wasn't as bad as I thought it would be. One key may have been that we did not give her the pacifier to suck on indiscriminately (we didn't just pop it in whenever her mouth was empty). It was always available when she wanted it, but we actually offered it to her only when she was agitated and needed comforting."

#7 Taking the Bull By the Horns

"Well I decided to take the bull by the horns and go cold turkey on weaning my eight-month-old. I decided it would be best to do this over a long weekend since he'd be back with his nanny the next week. I put him to bed at his usual time. He cried for about ten minutes, for which I was in and out. I picked him up but he kept trying to get out of my arms, so I left the room and he fell asleep in a few minutes. I couldn't believe it! He woke up and whimpered for a few minutes during the night but then fell back asleep! The next two days were similar, but then he just stopped waking at night. I don't know if its coincidence or not, but he is sleeping much, much better without it. I think that every baby is different and what works for some babies certainly won't work for others, but thank God we are now dummy free. Best of luck to anyone who is thinking of weaning."

#8 Good Ole Peer Pressure

"My six-year-old came home from kindergarten crying one day after another child made fun of her for sucking her thumb on the playground. She had fallen down and to stop from crying, she instinctively stuck her thumb right in there. She told me that she tried not to suck her thumb at school and wondered if she was the only one her age who still sucked her thumb. I reassured her, but also seized the opportunity to say that if she was ready to stop, I was ready to help her. She took me up on it, and we used socks on her hand at night and a charting system, and before the school year was done, so was her thumb sucking!"

#9 Cutting the Cord

"Around nine months, I took the binky away during the day. After a bit of fussiness, that went fine. Then I removed it for naptime. After three days of so-so naps, we were fine again. We then cut the cord at bedtime. We had two horrible nights, and then it was all over."

#10 Santa's Little Helper

"We actually *just* got our three-and-a-half-year-old off of the paci. We rounded them all up on Christmas Eve and told him that we were leaving them for Santa to take to little babies who needed them, and that Santa would leave an extra little toy for him. It actually worked really well—he only half-heartedly asked for them twice, and hasn't looked back since."

#11 Big Boys Don't Cry…for their paci

"My son was two when we took it away cold turkey. He was only using it during naps and at night, but we thought it was time to break the habit. We had just had a baby, so we told him big boys don't use pacifiers, only babies do and that was it. He's never asked for it again."

#12 Binky Fairy

"We started talking with our son about the fact that the pacifier fairy comes and takes binkies from big boys to give to babies, leaving presents for the big boy when he was about three. He has a baby brother, so this made sense to him. He

Turning Fear into Hope

also saw a TV show that talked about the tooth fairy, which also made the concept (particularly the gift part) more interesting to him. He used his pacifier for sleep only; we had just moved him into a big boy bed, so the pacifier was next on the agenda. The fairy came and left him a new truck to play with. Every time he asked about the binky, we reminded him about the fairy and the truck. Soon it was all forgotten."

Mommy Liza says:

I hear more success stories from parents who help their children cut out rather than cut back on pacifier use. Two moms from my playgroup decided to wean their children from the pacifier. One mom chose to slowly reduce her child's pacifier use over time, and the child is still using the pacifier a year and a half later. The other one told her child the pacifier fairy took the paci, and after a few difficult days, the habit was broken for good.

Sucking Secret #10:

The key to success is to hang in there and know that the torture is only temporary. Lots of others have done it before, and you too will survive.

Step 11

Dealing with the Aftermath: Alternative soothing techniques

A landmark study from the *Journal of the American Medical Association* showed that babies who sucked the pacifier were just as fussy as babies who hardly used it. Of course, we can't assume from this study that the pacifier is not a good soothing tool. Certainly our own research and personal experience shows that it is a great soothing tool! But what we can learn from this study is that parents of babies who don't suck the pacifier have successfully found other techniques to soothe their babies just as much as the pacifier would. There is hope! Just remember, you can teach your child alternate soothing techniques, but don't expect that you'll be able to eliminate his stress entirely. After all, stress is part of life, it's just about how you manage it.

Here are some tips on dealing with "post-sucking stress disorder" to ultimately stay pacifier and thumb sucking-free:

#1 Swaddling and Rocking

Parents can swaddle infants who were weaned from the pacifier in the first few months of life. They can also use swaddling as a distraction technique to prevent ever needing the pacifier or the thumb in the first place. Rocking can be used at any age, and bigger children can get the same sensation from a rocking chair or even a car ride.

#2 Bathing

A warm bath can be calming for practically anyone. Of course, you can't suddenly bathe your child in the middle of a meltdown at the grocery store, but at the end of the day it can have a nice, soothing effect. You could even bathe your little one more often during the transition period just to take the edge off.

#3 Music

Singing and soft music will always be the gold standard for helping your baby or child relax.

Dr. Sumi says:

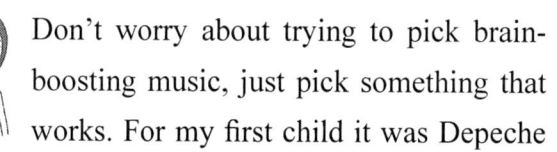

Don't worry about trying to pick brain-boosting music, just pick something that works. For my first child it was Depeche Mode starting at week three, and for my second one, it was and still is my own voice. I fear the day she realizes that I really can't carry a tune!

#4 Massage

For infants and any toddler who can sit still long enough, massage is a great tool for relaxation. You certainly don't have to have a degree in massage therapy, but there are parenting classes on massage (perhaps through your local hospital). The key is to calm your baby or child with the power of your touch. You can apply a little bit of baby oil and use slow and gentle strokes. Anything more than gentle strokes might not be appropriate for this age group without special training. You can intensify the calming effect with soft music or calming words as you massage.

#5 Extra Hugs

Along the lines of the unplug-and-hug weaning technique, you can continue to hug your child more frequently during the transition time as positive reinforcement. It can also help distract him every time he might ask for a pacifier or attempt to suck a thumb. This is a great strategy for any developmental phase.

#6 Help Your Child Communicate

Back to the original question, why does an infant use the pacifier? To soothe when stressed. What is stressful for an infant? Being hungry and tired. Therefore, if a child is able to communicate these feelings properly, this could greatly reduce their reliance on a pacifier or thumb, not to mention greatly reducing tantrums when they get older. You can help toddlers and preschoolers identify their feelings and talk about them.

Dealing with the Aftermath

Dr. Ruby says:

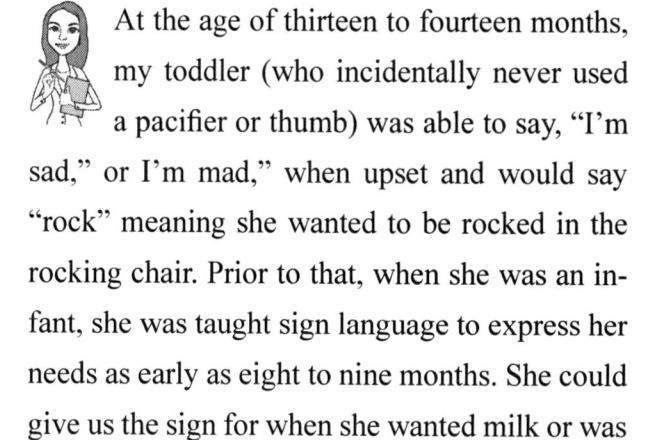

At the age of thirteen to fourteen months, my toddler (who incidentally never used a pacifier or thumb) was able to say, "I'm sad," or I'm mad," when upset and would say "rock" meaning she wanted to be rocked in the rocking chair. Prior to that, when she was an infant, she was taught sign language to express her needs as early as eight to nine months. She could give us the sign for when she wanted milk or was tired. This level of expression is very satisfying for a child and reduces frustration.

#7 Books, Games, and Videos

Books and games are great ways to engage and distract children of all ages. While these are best used to prevent a big fuss or tantrum, they can also be helpful to shorten fussy spells even just by hearing your voice in a soothing tone reading or telling a story. A favorite TV show or video can serve as a distraction and also a reward for being pacifier/thumb-free.

#8 Exercise

Research shows that exercise can be used to treat depression and possibly anxiety in adults, so it makes sense that it could reduce stress in children. If nothing else, it is a great distraction and has numerous other health benefits. Along the lines of the you're-all-grown-up weaning approach, this transition period is a great time to learn a new skill like riding a tricycle or a bicycle to boost self-confidence. Also consider lessons to learn a new skill, like swimming (good for all ages), yoga, or dance, to use up any negative energy.

#9 Make Them First Priority

It may sound silly to think of making your children first priority, especially when you feel like you've already dedicated your entire life to them. However, sometimes the everyday duties of childrearing and earning a living to support them can get in the way of actually spending quality time together.

Dealing with the Aftermath

Mommy Liza says:

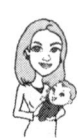

For adults, getting priority treatment can be soothing. Flying first class. Spending a day at the spa. The fine dining experience. There's nothing like it when your needs and wants are put first. Giving your kids priority treatment and a little pampering can be the ultimate soothing technique. I know parents who've cleared their schedules for a few days to focus on their children while they go through behavioral changes. Making your child your first priority and the focus of your attention can also provide an added sense of security and boost his self-esteem during times of change.

#10 Artwork

Drawing, coloring, clay art, building, and painting are other great ways to use up extra energy and create something positive. If your child is drawn to art projects, this is a perfect time to work on a slightly more challenging project together.

#11 Pet Therapy

Pets, both real and pretend, are incredible stress

relievers. It's amazing how a pet knows when you are feeling bad and will give you an extra snuggle or lick just to show you they care. We're not suggesting that you go out and buy your child a pet, though it's definitely an option. But if you have one, you can try to encourage a bond with your child by teaching him or her how to gently rub the pet and care for it. Even caring for a goldfish can be exciting for a child. If you don't have a pet, a pretend or stuffed pet that needs lots of hugs and attention might be just the distraction your child is craving.

#12 Sleeping Techniques

Don't fret about bedtime when the pacifier or thumb is finally gone, because there are other tried-and-true sleep techniques. The American Academy of Sleep Medicine produced a guideline on treatment of bedtime problems with techniques to help with falling asleep and to deal with late-night wake-ups. They point out that there is really no proof that one is better than the other (despite what your mother might tell you):

Dealing with the Aftermath

- unmodified extinction—this means put them to bed and let them cry it out.
- graduated extinction—this means letting them cry or self-soothe to sleep in specific time intervals. For example, let them cry for five minutes and then go back in the room to offer comfort. The next time, let them cry for ten minutes, etc.
- positive bedtime routines—this means setting a regular routine and time for sleep.
- delayed bedtime with removal from bed—this means putting them to bed closer to when they naturally appear sleepy. Positive bedtime routines can help have a consistent time of feeling sleepy each night. If they don't fall asleep within a certain time period, then they are removed from the bed (but not for play time). The process is then repeated.
- scheduled awakenings—this means waking them a little earlier than their typical night wakings (i.e., wake them before they wake you) and providing the usual

rocking, soothing, or feeding to put them back to bed

Sucking Secret #11:
Remember that the pacifier and thumb aren't the only successful ways to self-soothe. You can conquer those habits by teaching your child other techniques to cope during stressful situations.

Step 12

Learning from the Process: Help a friend and help yourself for future children

Congratulations! We've taken you through twelve weaning techniques, twelve success stories, and twelve alternative soothing techniques, and now we're finally at the twelfth step of the entire process. At this point, we hope that you have a good idea of what your plan is for your own little sucking addict, or that you've already put our techniques to the test! Keep in mind that there is a good chance you might have to use these strategies for a future child. We're not sure of the exact cause of family sucking traits, but it is likely a combination of genetic and environmental influences. Regardless, the lessons learned the first time around are often the key for the future.

If you feel you need additional information on specific topics, we have attached a resource list at the end of this book. Also, you can visit our Web site at www.pacifiersanonymous.com.

After you've gone through the rigorous process of weaning your child, it's natural to want to share some words of wisdom with other parents or caregivers—hence, the reason this book was written in the first place. We wanted to share our advice with you based on a combination of our unique perspectives of medical doctor, psychologist, and stay-at-home mom. Now it's your turn to take this information and pass it on.

As you've seen in this book, there are many ways to approach weaning; there are still some conflicting opinions about the health effects of sucking on the pacifier and thumb; and there are cultural variations on the subject too. Rather than pointing out a specific approach to someone else, perhaps you can take them briefly through how you got to where you are now. For example, we started the book acknowledging that parents ben-

Learning from the Process

efit and often enable sucking in their children. Next we talked about why babies like to suck in the first place and all of the potential good and bad health effects for each habit, including what various medical organizations recommend. We also discussed cultural trends and the results of our own survey. Next we explained how to figure out when the right time to wean is, which techniques have been used, and how to decide which technique might work best for your child. Finally we encouraged getting all the caregivers on the same team, shared success stories, and provided tactics for dealing with life after the beloved pacifier and thumb are out of the picture. Here we are full circle with step twelve, saying that the final step of the process is to use it again for the same or future children and share it with a friend. The twelve-step process is a tried-and-true technique that has had been successful for breaking numerous habits. The key is learning from it and using it again and again.

While the process can be challenging, when your child is finally pacifier/thumb-loose and fancy-free, it will all be worth it!

Sucking Secret #12:

Lessons learned from the process are what make it successful the next time around for you and for any friend in need.

The Twelve Steps and Twelve Sucking Secrets to Learn from Them

STEP 1	Admitting the Addiction: Who loves it more—you or your little one?	SUCKING SECRET #1	The pacifier or thumb can soothe the parents just as much as the child and can create a co-dependent habit. Just accept that and move on.
STEP 2	Knowledge Is Power: Understanding non-nutritive sucking and soothing	SUCKING SECRET #2	Despite which non-nutritive sucking theory you agree with, the bottom line is that infants are born with this survival instinct to suck and feed. Because this necessity creates pleasure, it can easily turn into a habit.
STEP 3	Making the Decision: Weighing the pros and cons	SUCKING SECRET #3	The main benefits to using the pacifier are pain relief, SIDS prevention, and even thumb-sucking prevention. The main risks are potential effects on breastfeeding if started too early, dental problems, and ear infections. The thumb may help with soothing but can cause dental problems and thumb deformities. Choose your vice and suck wisely!

STEP 4	Appreciating Differences: Cultural perspectives	SUCKING SECRET #4	Parents have been pacifying their babies for thousands of years with a variety of different objects. The popularity of the pacifier has had its ups and downs, and there are definitely cultural trends. Urban societies use the pacifier and thumb more than their rural counterparts who typically breastfeed more. This could be a case of the artificial versus human pacifier.
STEP 5	Turning to Others: A survey of what parents think	SUCKING SECRET #5	Pacifier use tends to start earlier but also ends earlier. Thumb use starts later but ends later. Many different weaning techniques can be used for pacifier suckers, with cold turkey being the most common, while thumb sucking usually stops naturally.
STEP 6	Getting Ready for the Big Day: Deciding when to make a clean break	SUCKING SECRET #6	Determine what motivates your little one to suck and assess any stressors in the environment. Know your limits. If you are having an extremely difficult time with weaning, or if you think it may be related to something else going on in your life, you can always ask for help.

STEP 7	Making a List: What weaning techniques have other parents used?	SUCKING SECRET #7	There are many great techniques for weaning, but don't be afraid to be creative and make up your own version. You can even use a few approaches together.
STEP 8	Choosing the Technique and Timing: What's best for you and your child	SUCKING SECRET #8	Remember to be realistic about your parenting style and practical about the timing, use positive reinforcement, and avoid power struggles. This will allow you to be consistent and effective with whichever method you choose.
STEP 9	Getting the Sponsors On Board: A united front	SUCKING SECRET #9	It is important to get the other sponsors/caregivers on board and make sure that everyone in the child's environment is doing the same thing.
STEP 10	Turning Fear into Hope: Success stories	SUCKING SECRET #10	The key to success is to hang in there and know that the torture is only temporary. Lots of others have done it before, and you too will survive.
STEP 11	Dealing with the Aftermath: Alternative soothing techniques	SUCKING SECRET #11	Remember that the pacifier and thumb aren't the only successful ways to self-soothe. You can conquer those habits by teaching your child other techniques to cope during stressful situations.
STEP 12	Learning from the Process: Help a friend and help yourself for future children	SUCKING SECRET #12	Lessons learned from the process are what make it successful the next time around for you and for any friend in need.

Resources

While professional experience is the backbone of this book, we certainly don't expect you to just take our word for it. We firmly believe that you should see the research we used as background. Of course, we didn't include every single study or article in the field, but we wanted to give you a summary of the most recent literature with the hope that you can look further into topics you find interesting. We begin with some helpful parenting Web sites and resources.

PARENTING WEB SITES

Familydoctor.org. Pacifiers: Benefits and Risks. http://familydoctor.org/online/famdocen/home/children/parents/infants/956.html
American Academy of Pediatrics. AAP Parenting Corner. http://www.aap.org/publiced/BR_Thumbs.htm.

American Academy of Pediatric Dentistry. AAPD fast facts 2007. http://www.aapd.org/media/FastFacts07.pdf.

JAMA Patient Page. Pacifiers and Breastfeeding. http://jama.ama-assn.org/cgi/reprint/286/3/374?maxtoshow=&HITS=10&hits=10&RESULTFORMAT=&fulltext=pacifier+patient+page&searchid=1&FIRSTINDEX=0&resourcetype=HWCIT.

Pediatrics for Parents. Vol 25, issues 7-8, pages 12-13. http://www.pedsforparents.com.

Zero to Three www.zerotothree.org

HEALTH EFFECTS

Sexton S, Natale R. Risks and benefits of pacifiers. Am Fam Physician. 2009 Apr 15;79(8):681-685.

American Academy of Pediatrics Subcommittee on Management of Acute Otitis Media. Diagnosis and management of acute otitis media. Pediatrics 2004;113(5):1451-65.
American Academy of Pediatrics, Task Force on Infant Sleep Position and Sudden Infant Death Syndrome. Changing concepts of sudden infant death syndrome: implications for infant sleeping environment and sleep position. Pediatrics 2000;105(3):650-6.

Center for Health Environment and Justice Bisphenol A Leaching from Popular Baby Bottle Is Your Baby's Bottle Potentially Harmful? http://www.chej.org/BPA_Website.htm

Community Paediatrics Committee, Canadian Paediatric Society (CPS)

Paediatrics & Child Health 2003; 8(8), 515-519. Reference No. CP03-01. Reaffirmed February 2009.
Davidson L. Thumb and finger sucking. Pediatr Rev. 2008; 29: 207-208.

Gartner LM, Morton J, Lawrence RA, Naylor AJ, O'Hare D, Schanler RJ, Eidelman AI. Breastfeeding and the use of human milk. Pediatrics 2005 Feb;115(2):496-506.

Hauck FR, Omojokun OO, and Siadaty MS. Do pacifiers reduce the risk of sudden infant death syndrome? A meta-analysis. Pediatrics. 2005; 116(5):716-723

Institute for Clinical Systems Improvement. Diagnosis and treatment of otitis media in children. http://www.icsi.org/otitis_media/diagnosis_and_ treatment_of_otitis_media_in_children_2304.html.

Marter A, Agruss, JC. Pacifiers: an update on use and misuse. J Spec Pediatr Nurs, 2007; 12(4):278-85.

North Stone K, Fleming P, Golding J. Pacifier use and morbidity in the first six months of life. Pediatrics. 1999; 103(3):E34.

North Stone K, Fleming P, Golding J. Sociodemographic associations with digit and pacifier sucking at 15 months of age and possible associations with infant infection. Early Hum Dev. 2000; 60(2):137-48.

O'Connor NR, Tanabe KO, Siadaty MS, Hauck FR. Pacifiers and breastfeeding: a systematic review. Arch Pediatr Adolesc Med. 2009 Apr;163(4):378-82.

Pinelli J, Symington A. Non-nutritive sucking for promoting physiologic stability and nutrition in preterm infants. Cochrane Database Syst Rev 2005;(4):CD001071.

Shotts L, McDaniel DM, Neely R. The impact of prolonged pacifier use on speech articulation: a preliminary investigation. Contemp Issues Commun Sci Disord. 2008; 35: 72-75.

US Consumer Product Safety Commision. CPSC Releases Study on Phthalates in Teethers, Rattles and Other Children's Products. http://www.cpsc.gov/cpscpub/prerel/prhtml99/99031.html

US Consumer Product Safety Commision. Requirements for Pacifiers, 16 C.F.R. Part 1511. Retrieved September 10, 2008. http://www.cpsc.gov/BUSINFO/regsumpacifier.pdf

Warren JJ, Bishara SE, Steinbock KL, Yonezu T, Nowak AJ. Effects of oral habits' duration on dental characteristics in the primary dentition. J Am Dent Assoc 2001;132(12):1685-93.

Zempsky WT, Cravero JP. Relief of pain and anxiety in pediatric patients in emergency medical systems. Pediatrics 2004; 114(5): 1348-56.

Barbosa C, Vasquez S, Parada MA, et al. The relationship of bottle feeding and other sucking behaviors with speech disorder in Patagonian preschoolers. BMC Pediatr. 2009 Oct 21;9(1):66.

Resources

HISTORICAL PERSPECTIVE

Anonymous. *New York Times*, June 30, 1909

Gale CR, Martyn CN. Dummies and the health of Hertfordshire infants, 1911-1930. Soc Hist Med.1995; 8(2):231-55.
Golubewa EL, Shulejkina KV, Vainstein II. The development of reflex and spontaneous activity of the human fetus during embryogenesis. Obstet Gynecol [USSR] 1959; 3:59-62.

How Products Are Made: Volume 7. 2007 Advameg Inc. Retrieved September 10, 2008 http://www.madehow.com/Volume-7/Pacifier.html.

Levin S. Dummies. S Afr Med J, 1971; 45(9):237-40. Winter GB. Problems involved with the use of comforters. Arch Dis Child. 2002; 87(2):170.

Pedley TF. The Rubber Teat and Deformities of the Jaws, Dental Record, 1907; 27: 176-77

King FT. Feeding and Care of Baby. London, 1923.
Sears, Roebuck & Company. *Sears, Roebuck Catalog* [Brochure] Chicago, IL: 1902.

CULTURAL PERSPECTIVES

Caglar E, Larsson E, Andersson EM, Hauge MS, Ogaard B, Bishara S, Warren J, Noda T, Dolci GS. Feeding, artificial sucking habits, and malocclusions in 3-year-old girls in different regions of the world. J Dent Child (Chic). 2005; 72(1):25-30.

Farsi NM, Salama FS. Sucking habits in Saudi children: prevalence, contributing factors and effects on the primary dentition. Pediatr Dent, 1997; 19(1): 28-33.

Giovannini M, Banderali G, Radaelli G, Carmine V, Riva E, Agostoni C. Monitoring breastfeeding rates in Italy: national surveys 1995 and 1999. Acta Pædiatrica. 2003; 92(3):357-363.

Hamlyn B, Brooker S, Oleinikova K, Wands S. Infant Feeding 2000. BMRB International. 2002

Hasunen K. Infant Feeding in Finland 2000, Reports of Ministry of Social Affairs and Health 2001; Vol. 12: p. 1236-2115.

Resources

International Institute for Population Sciences (IIPS) and Macro International. 2007. National Family Health Survey (NFHS-3), 2005-6, India: Key Findings. Mumbai: IIPS.

Nelson EA, Yu LM, Williams S, and International Child Care Practices Study Group Members. International Child Care Practices study: Breastfeeding and pacifier use. J Human Lactation. 2005; 21:3: 289-295.

Sarkar S, Chowdhury KS, Mukherjee MM. Prevalence of thumb sucking in children of Calcutta. J Indian Soc Pedod Prev Dent.1992; 10(1):33-6.

Tepora E, Nurtitila A, Sairanen S, Riihelä J. Breastfeeding of babies in Vantaa 1997. Sosiaali- ja terveydenhuollon toimialan julkaisuja (Report). 1999; C:14.

UNICEF. Progress for Children: A World Fit for Children Statistical Review. Number 6, 2007.

PSYCHOLOGY OF SUCKING

Bakwin H. Thumb- and finger-sucking in children. J Pediatr, 1948; 32:99-101. And Ozturk M, Ozturk OM. Thumbsucking and falling asleep. Br J Med Psychol, 1977; 50:95-103.

Freud S. The Origin and Development of Psychoanalysis. First published in Am J Psychology, 1910; 21:181-218.

Larsson EF, Dahlin KG. The prevalence and the etiology of the initial dummy- and finger- sucking habit. Am J Orthod. 1985; 87(5):432–435.

Slaughter WC, Cordes CK. Covert maternal deprivation and pathological sucking behavior. Am J Psychiatry, 1977; 134:1152-3.

Warren JJ, Levy SM, Nowak AJ, Tang S. Non-nutritive sucking behaviors in preschool children: a longitudinal study. Pediatr Dent. 2000; 22(3):187-91.

BREASTFEEDING

Aarts C, Hörnell A, Kylberg E, Hofvander Y, Gebre-Medhin M. Breastfeeding patterns in relation to thumb sucking and pacifier use. Pediatrics 1999;104(4):e50.

American Academy of Family Physicians. Breastfeeding (position paper). http://www.aafp.org/online/en/home/policy/policies/b/breastfeedingpositionpaper.html. Accessed March 14, 2008.

Beck TR, Combs AA, Eversmann KD, Serrell B. *Kids! 200 Years of Childhood.* Hanover, New Hampshire: University Press of New England;1999.

Betrán AP, de Onís M, Lauer JA, Villar J. Ecological study of effect of breast feeding on infant mortality in Latin America. BMJ. 2001; 323:303.

Center for Disease Controls and Prevention. Breastfeeding Report Card – United States 2009.

http://www.cdc.gov/breastfeeding/data/report_card2.htm. Accessed December 23, 2009.

de Onis M. The optimal duration of exclusive breastfeeding: RHL commentary (last revised: 11 November 2002). The WHO Reproductive Health Library, No 9, Update Software Ltd, Oxford, 2006. Retrieved September 8, 2008. www.rhlibrary.com.

El-Zanaty F, Way AA. Nutritional Status, prevalence of anemia and micronutrient supplementation. Demographic and Health Survey 2000; 163-170.

Empowering women to breastfeed. Guidelines for action Report 1995; Retrieved on September 10, 2008.

Gartner LM, Morton J, Lawrence RA, Naylor AJ, O'Hare D, Schanler RJ, Eidelman AI. Breastfeeding and the use of human milk. Pediatrics 2005 Feb;115(2):496-506.

Howard CR, Howard FM, Lanphear B, Eberly S, deBlieck EA, Oakes D, Lawrence RA. Randomized clinical trial of pacifier use and bottle-feeding or cupfeeding and their effect on breastfeeding. Pediatrics. 2003 Mar;111(3):511-8.

International Lactation Consultant Association (ILCA). Clinical guidelines for the establishment of exclusive breastfeeding. Raleigh (NC); International Lactation Consultant Association (ILCA).2005 Jun. 28

Joanna Briggs Institute. Early childhood pacifier use in relation to breastfeeding, SIDS, infection, and dental malocclusion. Nurs Stand 2006; 20:52-5.

Kramer MS, Barr RG, Dagenais S, et al. Pacifier use, early weaning, and cry/fuss behavior. JAMA 2001;286:322-6.

Kutlu R, Marakoglu K. Evaluation of initiating, continuing and weaning time of breastfeeding. Marmara Medical Journal. 2006; 19(3):121-126.

Levy SM, Slager SL, Warren JJ, Levy BT, Nowak AJ. Associations of pacifier use, digit sucking, and child care attendance with cessation of breastfeeding. J Fam Pract. 2002 May; 51(5):465.

Li R, Zhao Z, Mokdad A, Barker L, Grummer-Strawn L. Prevalence of breastfeeding in the United States: the 2001 National Immunization Survey. Pediatrics. 2003; 111:1198 –1201.

Rogers IS, Emmett PM, Golding J. The incidence and duration of breastfeeding. Early Hum Dev. 1997; 49(suppl): S45-S74.

Vallenas C, Savage F. World Health Organization review: Evidence for the 10 steps to successful breastfeeding. 1998.

UNICEF. Progress for Children: A World Fit for Children Statistical Review. Number 6, 2007.

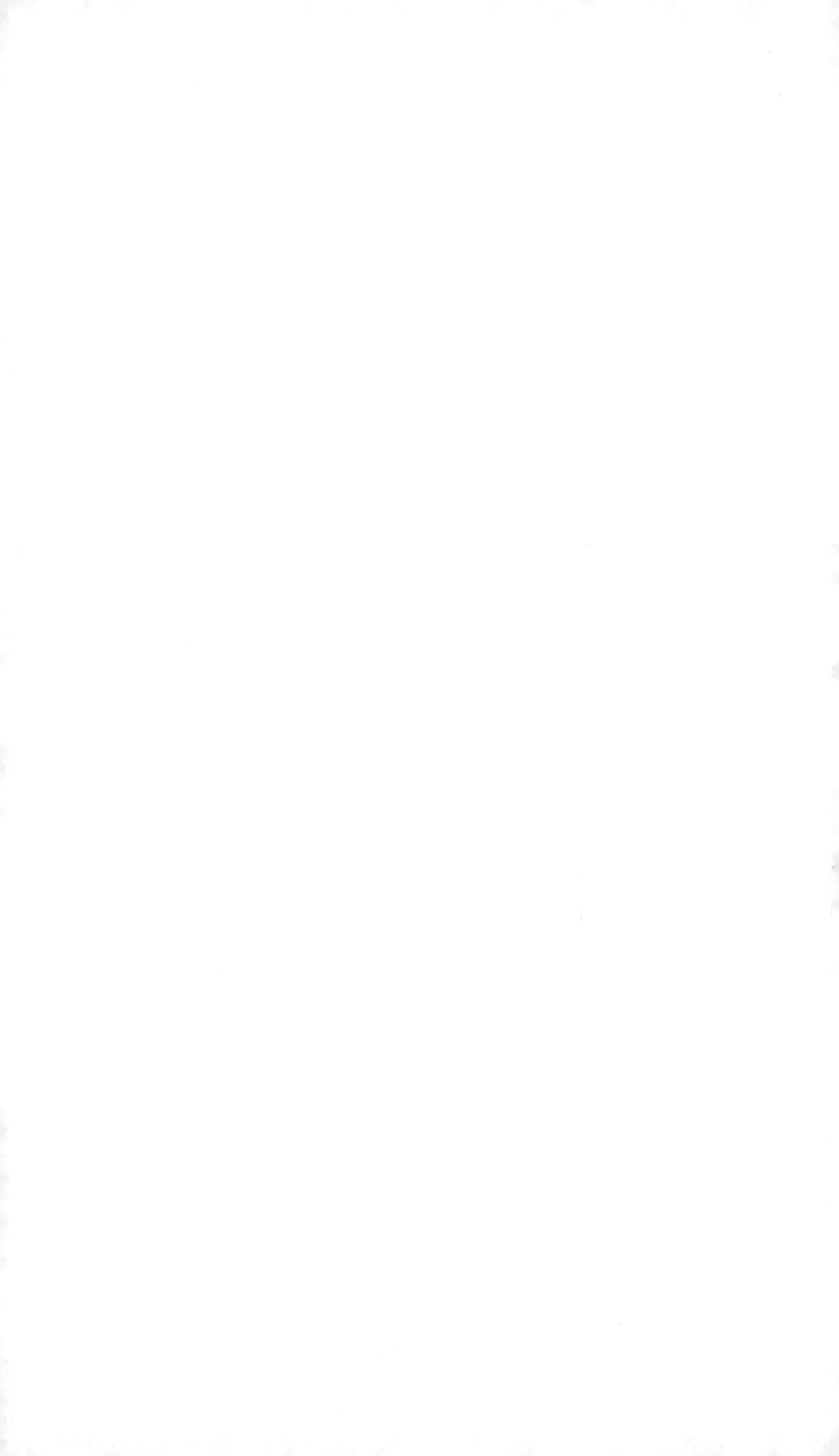

LaVergne, TN USA
20 February 2011
217224LV00004B/3/P